AVOIDANCE, DRUGS, HEARTBREAK & DOGS

Also by Jordan Stephens

The Missing Piece

AVOIDANCE, DRUGS, HEARTBREAK & DOGS

Jordan Stephens

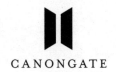

CANONGATE

Dedicated to Spike the God

First published in Great Britain in 2024
by Canongate Books Ltd, 14 High Street, Edinburgh EH1 1TE

canongate.co.uk

1

British Library Cataloguing-in-Publication Data
A catalogue record for this book is available on
request from the British Library

ISBN 978 1 83885 808 7

Typeset in Sabon by Palimpsest Book Production Ltd,
Falkirk, Stirlingshire

Printed and bound by CPI Group (UK) Ltd,
Croydon CR0 4YY

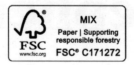

MIX
Paper | Supporting
responsible forestry
FSC® C171272
www.fsc.org

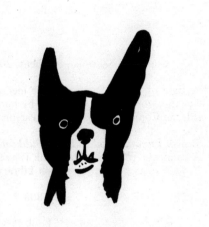

'There are only two things promised in life . . . change and death.'

Uber driver

CONTENTS

Preface

Dear Reader,

I've chosen to write this book mainly in the present tense. I want you to accompany me out of the shadows. Enhance the journey. Aid the adventure. So for clarity. It's important to me that I'm honest about my journey. Even me at my most deluded. I've written this for the heartbreakers and the heartbroken. It's all my own experience. I'm not interested in sanitising anything. Everyone's got a shadow – that's something I can say confidently. This hypermoralistic outlook on society, or the belief that people can be infallible, is fucking ridiculous. And the reality of growing up as a boy, becoming a man, in this culture of sex, money and murder is not pretty. We have been indoctrinated. Stripped of ourselves at times. And there's deeper we can go too. It's discouraged to air the truth. Male minds are fucked by this point. We're burdened by a fear of vulnerability and a desire to fuck everything. Again, ridiculous and provocative but true. And we're not going to be able to evolve if we can't move past denial. We're going to start in the mud and move up.

This book isn't supposed to be prescriptive. It's not supposed to be knowing or aware. It's a heady monologue. A chaos mind journey in a memory vehicle. A shared wince. Self-harm at times too, maybe. I'm not averse to hurting myself for entertainment. Someone once asked me how I'd want to be remembered. I said, 'As the boy who grew.'

Jordan
April 2024

1

Wired

I started eating explosives before I could spell my name. Devoured bombs before breakfast. Picked the wires out of my teeth. Looked like I was smiling. You're supposed to explode as a kid. Keep the energy moving. Communicate that core position. But in this country you're encouraged to eat fury. Lips pursed. Remain immovable. People wait too long to let their tongues tick, so it becomes rage. I swallowed these bombs and they exploded into my existence as I got older. The clouds formed into self-destruction, addiction. My attention scattered. Because I'd left it too long. And because of fights beyond my control. When I was diagnosed with ADHD at 15, I became another statistic. Another young boy from a low-income, single-parent household who can't concentrate.

I ate the bombs and they left a void. As well as a desire to escape. And so, naturally, I worked harder than anybody my age as a teenager. Became successful young. Tried to fill that void with attention. A common trait of the young and famous. The desire to escape. I did my best to earn money as a teenager to alleviate the pressure on my mum. We had very little. But the emotional world doesn't care about the physical one. My unprocessed feelings were around the corner waiting. Regardless of how 'well I did'. I had everything and nothing at the same time. I wasn't poor enough to be a criminal but I wasn't rich enough to be one either. A freelance, self-employed inventor. Writer, performer, multi-hyphen clown. Millennial sleazeball. I'd done well enough to lend my family money. That money also meant I had time. And there was a time when that time attacked me.

But I've learnt that anger and love aren't opposing forces. They've got to balance to exist. All emotions have to be processed. Anger is knowing what I deserve on my plate. And love is delicious. But seeing and accepting the healthy and unhealthy strands of my personality for what they are has not been an easy journey. Wouldn't be worth it if it was.

Funny how one moment can change an entire life. In my case, that was being left by a girlfriend after telling her I'd been unfaithful. A girlfriend I was convinced I was in love with. I figured it's worth writing about. Because this shit happens all the time. But I don't hear enough about it. Not from this angle anyway.

To find my way towards a healthy relationship with anger I had to overcome obstacles. Namely my parents.

I'm closer to my mum and dad than I have been in a long time. Shit had to change. I had to grow up and confront the gods. They're worried about this book. Concerned with their own legacy. Usually an author's parents pass before they dissect them. I'm not waiting that long. And I believe, now we're closer, that they understand. They get that whatever I write might help someone else.

It's about creating something that could outlive you or me. Words are forever.

When I look into my mum's seaside eyes – blue and green – I can see her love for me. And for the world. I can see what she's had to work through, and how hard she is on herself. Except I don't feel it squeezing my belly like I used to. I feel separate. Which is a good thing. It's hard watching her stay afloat at times. Burdened by distance in her youth from her own parents. Bullied by a system she's spent her life opposing. Her heart is certainly in the right place. Always on hand to help and encourage. Puts herself second a lot. Which is decent in moderation. But it's one trait I've learnt to ditch.

Without my mum, I wouldn't be who I am today. A worrier and a wonderer. A proponent of going your own way. Separating from the herd.

When I hang out with my dad and his new family, I catch him staring out the corner of my eye. Like he's taking me in. Marvelling at his creation. He too is a survivor. Of fucking everything. And I feel that now. I'm soothed by it. As I grow older. As the rings add up. So does my love for him. But it's not been easy. And I've needed to be honest to move past the anger. There's so much about him I still don't know.

2

My Mum Killed Our
Neighbour's Dog

My mum killed our neighbour's dog. When I was 16. It was an accident. Dog had it coming unfortunately. He was an idiot. Was unable to run and face forwards at the same time. I love dogs but sometimes you have to be realistic. I tried to warn the owner's son, Joel. Told him to be careful. I said you can't keep chasing him around the mews if he's incapable of looking ahead. I really stressed how anti-survival that trait was. This tiny little black dog. Could have been a toy. Ran around like he'd been wound up that morning. Like he had a silver winder on his back. We were looking after my dad's old dog, Narco, at the time. Big white Alsatian. If our door was open, as it often was in this mews, this little hamster excuse-for-a-canine would bolt inside. Sprint circles around Narco, who would just look up at me as if to say, 'What the fuck is this thing?'

The mews we used to live in was an unsolved Rubik's cube. Every neighbour a new assortment of clashing colours. It led from the street in a backwards L-shape, with most houses hidden from view. That didn't stop people wandering down at night though. Trying to steal a bike. Trying to wank each other off on the bench backed into the corner. Only the older couple at number 1 lived through more iterations of mews occupants. My mum and I weren't even there that long. A few years. We rubbed bricks with all types of folk. Matt, a masseuse who collected samurai swords. His partner Flora, a reflexologist who once cured my headache by rubbing my little toe. Emily and Jason. Jason was an ex-rugby player turned border police officer. Told me how many times people had tried to stab him. I could hear Emily crying through my bedroom wall when they found out he had a brain tumour. Dan and Sarah had a dangerous domestic. Word on the mews was he broke her foot. She called the police. He ended up being pepper-sprayed to the ground and arrested. I slept through the whole thing. Alexis and Iris. In a permanent state of yoga. Probably had carpets on the walls. Herbal tea only. Topi, a tall, leggy, model-type woman who lived alone. Sometimes men would turn up looking smug. Rarely would we see them again. After they left, that was. Her killing extended only to fashion. The most memorable, however, was easily Joel and his mum. The dead dog being a big reason. But even outside that. They were still there when we left.

Joel was a bizarre boy. Was a goth from the age of 7. Had this mosh-pit black fringe. Always wanted to play football with me. Didn't say much. Seemed a little out of sync with his own body. His mum, Julia, was also gothic. Had a Halloween vibe about her. Spoke like she was hiding something in her cheeks. Smiled every now and again. Walked like a troubled puppet. Caught a couple of shifty-looking men stood outside their place once. My personal highlight was when Julia forgot her keys. Joel was so fast asleep in the bed upstairs that he couldn't hear her banging. Couldn't hear her shouting his name. Was in some kind of coma. I had to get the ladder out, climb up to the top window to check he was alive. I stood silently for a second. The gothy prince was out cold. Knocking the glass did the trick. Panic over.

There was another layer to the dog story. Taints the giggles, to be honest. He was a substitute. A distraction. Joel's dad had killed himself a couple of months before. Overdosed. Another untenable soul back to spirit. Julia took it pretty hard. Joel turned into a garden gnome. Hard as stone. I'd pass the football to him. He'd trap it under his foot, look at me and say, 'My dad's dead.'

I'd say, 'I know.'

Then he'd pass the ball back.

There's usually an apology after. Maybe I did apologise. But grief's a riddle for a young heart. I was still a kid too. The mortality conundrum. Loss. Disappearance. Could quite easily be a trick. My instinct was to be casual. To respond as if he was asking the time. Didn't even ask him if he was ok. Just thought I'd be there when I could. Pass the ball to him. Didn't have much else to offer. I could have hugged him. Apologised some more. Some ways work. I didn't know any of the ways. Maybe I would have wanted to be hugged. At his age I didn't even think I could die. Genuinely remember feeling invincible. Like I could walk into the street and cars would avoid me.

One time I passed him the ball. He mistimed his feet. Stepped on it. Fell flat on his face. I'm talking nose into concrete. Straight gravity. Before I could even run to his aid, he was up. No complaints. Not even a wince. Breathed out, passed the ball back.

I'm guessing the dog was a life replacement. That's why it's such a shame it was hellbent on dying. Poor thing just wanted to run around. Get chased by Joel. Tongue wagging. Non-stop movement. My mum pulled her car around to the front of the mews. Car wasn't moving but the engine was on. Joel chased the dog round the corner. The dog ran full pelt underneath the static car and smashed its head on something underneath it. The radiator or something. Fuck knows. Something hot. It popped back out the other side. Ran back into the house and collapsed in Julia's arms. Couldn't have written it. Fortunately Ralph, one of the older neighbours, saw the whole thing. Julia ran back out of the mews with the dog in her arms and my mum drove her to doggy hospital. Mum says Ralph got in too and he was halfway through an ice cream. The dog died on the way there.

Julia wore all black for a month at least. She might have worn black for longer than she had the dog. Joel didn't say much. Maybe he blamed himself. Guilt. Another adolescent Everest. She knocked at our door one evening. Everything in our living room was turquoise. Crystals lined all shelves. Incense lingered. The timing couldn't have been worse. I was really fucking stoned. Two thirds of the way through a chocolate croissant and halfway through an episode of *Futurama*. My mum opened the door and Julia immediately threw her arms around her. Sobbing. Smelt of alcohol. Kept on saying, 'It's not your fault. It's not your fault.'

I didn't even have to see my mum's face to know her

expression. She would have had seven teeth in her tongue. We knew it wasn't my mum's fault. We had got over the death very quickly. Sounds mean but, honestly, if you'd met this dog.

I was trying so desperately hard not to laugh. Pure evil. Wouldn't dream of it. And yet I couldn't even relax my lips for loose pastry. Out of fear. The back of my throat was vibrating. It was nervous laughter too. Like laughing at a funeral. The more you think about not laughing, the more it hits your belly. Tears were beginning to form around my eyes. I did everything to avoid catching my mum's gaze. I felt bad for Julia though. Genuinely. This was a lot. I just wish I wasn't stoned.

They ended up getting another dog quite quickly. This one was a little bigger and could run looking forwards. Not that it had much of an opportunity to. It was in a harness and on a lead the entire time. I kept wanting to tell Joel that this was a different dog. This one could run facing the right way. But I never did. Poor thing was being punished for a life it never knew. The beginning of a toxic cycle.

3

A Year *After* I Fucked Up:
Part One

Weekday morning in 2018. I'm 28. In the city. I've got an open-plan situation in my flat. Big, tinted balcony doors. I can see out but others can't see in. That's what they told me anyway. The tint tends to steal tone. Outside is always brighter than what makes it through. Opposite those doors are windows with Venetian blinds. That's the vibe for the flat. Blinds you can twizzle open. These ones often get shut because the view is into the car park and other people's lives. One guy has a fuck-off projector and I'm fuming about it. Unbelievably high definition. Another guy has a big skinny dog. He's always in his pants. Has a nice car. My friend Lucy lives diagonally across. Most days she sits with a spliff in her hand. Elegantly deathscrolling. Making herbal teas. Moves her lips when her boyfriend's there. I haven't got much to do today. My girlfriend left early. Couldn't leave her cats for too long. Got to feed those psychopaths. I'm a few months into owning a dog. He's kind of special, I think. Not like other dogs. Incredibly chill. Could be Buddhist. In the drawer next to the fridge I keep all types of shit. This includes some rolled-up tinfoil protecting three or four freeze-dried magic mushrooms. Bought them off my friend round the corner. He's an enthusiast. Makes house music in his spare time. Has a beautiful child. Says these shrooms are from Scotland. Says the United Kingdom is bettered only by Hawaii for magic mushroom birthing. Might be nice to have one. In some tea. Walk amongst nature. A little buzz to start the day. Could eat the whole lot and see if I can speak dog. Nah, just the one. A little tickle.

By the time I get to the park I should start feeling the effects. I wind down towards it. Dog on lead. Kensal Rise is typically invasive. Smoggy intersections. Privileged prams. Dystopian estates. A cauldron of culture, like so many corners of London. People are three wage brackets and two languages away from their next-door neighbours. It quietens down a bit at this time in the morning. Most people are at work. In West London especially, late-morning weekday walks are reserved almost exclusively for failed artists. Gazing at ducks, hoping for inspiration. Throwing bread in battered leather jackets. I get to the gates of the park. Let my dog off the lead. The park is ideal. Big green in the middle perfect for chucking balls. Although I have to be careful. My dog's a ball thief. A good one too. I've been known to carry spares. There was a guy here hitting golf balls once. Pretty reckless. Potential dog killer. There are shrubs and secret pathways. There's even a little sandpit designated as a dog litter. Never have I seen a dog well-trained enough to position themselves there though. Elite dogs only.

I start to wash around the park slowly. Breathe in something nearer clean air. Starting to feel the effects a little. Noticing the shape of shadows. That's what I love most about psychedelics. Greeting beauty I usually take for granted. Feeling connected. That's what it's all about. Might stand on a bench. Trees really are breathtaking. And breathgiving. Standing people. Waving. Swimming in the wind. I'm kind of lost in it. I'm central to the path as it curves round. There is no race. I'm not competing in this moment. What a peaceful dissonance from everyday imbalance. I could raise my arms right now and glide. Do an aeroplane. I wonder if my dog's having a shit. Doesn't matter, it's all bushes around here. It's all leaves and ladybirds. Worse for the planet to put it in plastic anyway. Unless another dog walker sees it. Then it's a crime. Dog walkers can be awful snitches. Can't see any. Nothing happened then. For a moment my dog bounds past my line of vision and disappears into another rustle of leaves. Sounds like scrunching tinfoil. That's when another dog rounding the opposing corner grabs my attention. Bites it. I think it's a dog anyway. It's huge. A big grey dog a lot larger than mine. Like a wolf. The nearer I get, the more wolflike it becomes. This looks like a fucking wolf. It's moving very slowly. A few paces behind it, a figure appears. A woman. A short woman with an oversized dark blue cap. Facing the ground as she treads. As if she's surveying her own steps. This is definitely a wolf. Am I tripping? Surely I'd be pulsating for a hallucination of this nature. I'm about to greet a wolf. I'm full of air. Fucking fascinated. On a different day, I might just walk past. Tell someone about it later. Deliberate on it. Make it stranger. Yeah, yesterday I stroked a stray wolf. But today I'm craving clarity. I walk towards the lady. Pick the right words. I should ask what breed. Something normal.

'Excuse me, is this your wolf?'

Just came out. The woman lifts her head and meets my gaze. Headlights in the dog park. She's a lot shorter than me so she's looking up. Dark brown eyes, dark brown hair. Spanish-looking. Not sure if that's offensive. Tanned skin. She looks as if she's been walking this wolf all day. My enquiry hasn't fazed her at all. Totally nonplussed. Like she was expecting the question. After a couple of seconds, she replies.

'Yes. You know this wolf.'

4

Six Months *Before* I Fucked Up

I used to date a girl who told me she had a fear of babies crawling towards her. She was laid on my rug when she said that. Legs kicked in the air like a magazine shoot. My best mate thought it was hilarious. Hasn't let go of it. That was the first place I ever lived in on my own. Had this fuck-off window. Overlooked a railway. I'd look out the window every night in the hope I'd catch someone having sex. Some rear in the rear window. It was open plan. Literally nothing on the walls. Cheap sofa. Great neighbours. And this lingering scent of modernity that acted as a warm, stale reminder that London is over-crowded. New builds everywhere.

This girl was a glamour model. Messy blonde. Watery blue eyes. Western-male-gaze-type naughty when serious. Childlike when smiling. Showed a bit of gum under her top lip. Kind of posh, too, which was a bit disorientating. In fact, she was the face of the 'Save Page 3' campaign. Can't say I endorsed it. Told her that. She told me the paper would pay her a monthly retainer on top of flying her and her friends out on holiday to take a few pictures. Good deal. Not her fault we can't separate mind from

17

breast. Who was I kidding? Got a bit of power and started spilling my childhood inadequacy. I'd say things like 'you should pursue painting' as if my house was rigged with feminist spyware. In reality I figured her figure was enough. I learnt the hard and, in hindsight, fairly quick way that it wasn't.

One afternoon she asked me if her friend could stay the night with her. Her friend was also a glamour model. The text said 'three in a bed?' with a winky face after. No fucking way. No fucking way she means that. A prospect that frequented my adolescent dreams. Got to be a trap. I agreed. Neighbours rubbernecking as they turned up in leather. Short skirts at the least.

I felt like
the man
based off the reactions of
the men
nearby.

Her friend was Eastern European. Confidently brunette. Semi-aggressive brow. Big breasts.

In my mind I was backstroking through memories of being 14. Kissing Daisy in the cinema. Then ringing her the next day and finding out she was actually going to go for Jack. Having rumours spread about me at school that I had a small dick. I bet I fucking did. Walking to the bus stop by the high road with two girl mates of mine. Shrinking while they debated whose dick they were going to suck that night. Ramming desperation for that dick to be my own into the back of my head. Crumpling it up and shoving it into the same pocket of confusion that housed my intrigue for sexy desktop wallpapers of curvaceous actresses.

Quite quickly, I hit it off with her mate. Not even in a sexual way. She was direct. Knew what she wanted. Exposed male fragility, willingly. Men would just buy her things. We ended up getting lost in conspiracies. All of us tried watching a shitty film but the conversation meandered. Drunk on existentialism. Feeling tipsy too. The girl I was seeing was on a course of antibiotics so was off her face. After some time she decided to fuck things off and shove her mate in the spare room. Literally shove her. Threw my pet tiger in behind her. Cuddly toy.

When we got into my room she wanted to have sex. I was hesitant. She was more drunk than I was. I said no. She wouldn't take no for an answer. Said we'd have sex again so it didn't matter. She was sober enough to present herself. I figured her figure was enough.

It was visually stunning. Spiritually, less so. Curves, arches, rhythm. As if manifested from my own conditioned gaze. She watched herself in the mirror beside my bed. A mirror gifted to me by my neighbour. Told me I'd thank him later. My thoughts were toffee and inescapable. I struggled not to cum too quickly. It was as if being partially present accelerated the pleasure. She was driving. While on top of me she grabbed my throat. Sexy at first until she genuinely shut my windpipe. Couldn't even tell her to ease off. As legendary as it would be to die at the hands of a glamour model, I got on top to regain control/not die. And after I did, she sunk her claws in. Maybe in an attempt to erase that evening's misjudgements. She dug her nails into both shoulder blades and pulled downwards while her housemate spooned my tiger. It fucking hurt.

I really did want to be in the same cage as her. But my

back felt like a chalkboard. I asked her not to go so hard. She grunted a little, squealed even, and then did it again. With more force. I recoiled from beside her neck.

'STOP IT. You're hurting me!' I said.

Honestly, I like pain. And back scratches might even be the number-one most impressive sexual souvenir. But these nails were like little pocketknives and I hated it. Missionary continued. Then she grabbed my necklace. Like she was falling off a cliff. It wasn't a great necklace, but I still didn't want it ripped off my fucking neck. I liked it enough to not want it destroyed. She looked a little shocked that she'd pulled it off. I was angry. Jaw clenched, lips pursed kind of angry. Eyes shut, take-a-breath-in kind of angry. While having sex. I asked her as calmly as possible to give me the necklace. She placed it in my palm. I put it on my bedside table before silently resuming my hip motion.

*

I'm pretty sure my mum's bought me a necklace.

It's a friendly afternoon in Kensal Rise. I'm 27. Rays slicing through my Venetian blinds. My bedroom is mainly cream and white. Haven't got round to properly decorating yet. I've got one film poster up on the wall. It's for a French New Wave film called *Breathless*. Jean-Luc Godard. The first line of the film is 'After all, I'm an arsehole'. Studied it in college.

My mum's in the middle of the doorway and my hands are cupped. She's about to give me a gift. Another suggestion. Something hard to find. Something I haven't realised I like yet. These days each gift feels like a reminder to wake up. To open my eyes to her understanding of my future. I worry there's too much value in my reaction. My flat's a cokey sentence. There are hand marks on the walls where there should be more pictures. There've been beanbags with cigarette wounds bleeding beans onto the floor. I've got too many trainers. I've got a pair of Kanye West Nike Yeezys that are worth thousands. They don't mean much to me. But I am stepping away from my mother. I don't see her as much and my dreams are less weighty.

I thought my mum was 27 for ages. Turns out she gave birth to me when she was 31. Wanted to keep her stage age down. Friends got her fake cards and everything. I can't remember being shocked. It's totally in keeping with her attitude. She refuses even to be bound by time. She also wants me to play 'Should I Stay Or Should I Go Now?' by The Clash at her funeral. At least that's sorted. I don't think about her dying much. Don't want to. Maybe when I was a kid. I used to have this recurring nightmare that our council flat in Neasden would split in two, with each of us on either side, and just drift into space like a departing starship. I remember seeing the universe between us. Fortunately I didn't develop a fear of the night sky. Quite the opposite in fact. Even now I look for Orion's Belt and feel secure. Get buzzed at the sight of Betelgeuse. Probably quite unusual for a child to name their first tiger toy after a constellation. Cassiopeia. That tiger's seen a lot.

My mum's tall, but not short on opinions. I was born into protest. She hates the system. Used to wear a t-shirt with 'McShit' written on it. Hates the government. Amnesty posters everywhere. Believes in magic. We buried crystals on Hampstead Heath, by the Winnie-the-Pooh tree. I remember the warmth of a tiger's eye in my palm. Held it in my little hands to protect me. Drunk soya milk until it was genetically modified. Mostly vegetarian.

The first time I went to a birthday party at McDonald's I asked why the cheese was made of plastic. I wasn't allowed to be picky. I ate what I was given. I tried oysters before I was 10. Some of the relatives on my mum's side loved to live rich even if they were skint. Three-tuxedos-no-house kind of vibe. Revelled in etiquette.

My mum owns my tastebuds. She decided on them. She has good taste for the most part. Sometimes needlessly experimental. If I asked for a sandwich at the shop, she'd almost certainly find one with spinach and mango chutney in it. Sometimes a kid just wants cheese, know what I mean? She loves introducing me to new things. But as I've got older and formed my own opinions, her suggestive power has wavered.

She places a ball of tissue paper in my hand and looks up at me. Short red hair at the moment. Gymnastic brows. I pull the tissue paper apart and see a wolf staring back. A crystal wolf head hung with black lace. I would never wear this. I think she knows that I would never wear this but she wants me to.

'It's labradorite,' she says. 'Very hard to find actually . . .'
I bet.
'. . . took ages to arrive.'
I just can't imagine wearing a crystal necklace. I don't think I'm that guy. I'm more into gold and shit. I can imagine her wearing it.

'It wasn't cheap, you know.'

It's definitely a statement piece. Worthy of someone asking where it's from. Although sometimes a person will ask you a question to stop themselves from insulting you. This wolf's staring at me and I'm cast back to pulling up on an A-road next to a field somewhere just outside the city. We used to find fields a lot. Stick buttercups under our chins. Look up foxgloves in *Reader's Digest*. This was nighttime though, and a few of my mum's mates were there. Same ones who told me she was 27. We'd run into the fancy glow of a full moon and howl. Howl until our stomachs stretched. Let the lack of light eat our fury. We're lunatics.

'Ah, thank you. It's really cool.'

Genuinely trying to be enthusiastic. My mum pre-empts my underwhelm and assures me I will grow to understand it. Eyes flicker with disappointment. I will appreciate it when the time's right.

'No, honestly, I really like it. I'm not gonna wear it right now though.'

'Well, I just want you to know that it'll protect you. Labradorite is very powerful.'

I can only think of Labradors when she mentions the crystal. I love Labradors. Especially the chocolate ones. They don't know when to stop eating though. They can eat themselves to death – it's really sad. There's a little booklet with the necklace that I say I'm going to read. I place it all down on my table of things I like looking at and move the day along.

5

Five Months Before

It's my best friend Tai's birthday. Two thirds into spring. Sun walking away from winter's misery. I tell him I've arranged to meet up with this woman called Chloe who I said hi to at a club last week. He promotes the event with a buzz. He's stacked. Used to be my personal trainer. More like a brother now. Him and my ride-or-die, Jake. His smile and laughter are stimulants. Life's been sweet lately. Ever since I balanced on the back two legs of my dining chair. Gripped the edge of the chipped black dining table. Broke away from my ex. Wasn't clean but it feels like it. I do whatever I want now. I'm in my twenties with time, money and fuck-all responsibility. When I met this girl this other night I wasn't even drinking. Didn't feel like it. Did a French exit. Went home and ate pizza. All I do is take these Modafinil tablets I bought off the internet for my ADHD and think of a hundred new projects a day.

Tai recited a proverb recently. It wasn't verbatim. He's not great with words but he's great with heart. And the words have circled my mind like trotting horses ever since. He said, 'You know one of my favourite quotes ever. It's an old proverb actually. I think it's Native American or something. I want to be able to recite it to you properly but you know I'm shit with words.'

'Tell me it, you prick!'

'Alright . . . basically . . .'

Honestly, look this up after I say it, but basically . . . A guy is telling his son or grandson, whatever, and he says, inside us there are two wolves. At war. Fighting each other. One is anger, jealousy, resentment, guilt, envy, all of that shit. And the other wolf is joy, peace, love, generosity, truth and faith. All the good shit.

This must be word for word . . .

The kid looks up at him and says, 'But which wolf wins?' And the man replies by saying, 'The one you feed.'

Surely everyone's heard of this. I hadn't. Rung true. I looked it up and realised that its origins are unclear. In some spaces the 'two wolves' concept has reached parody. And apparently it's not even Native American. I fuck with the notion though. Feed the wolf fucked-up shit and what do I think's going to happen? I've got to start feeding the right wolf the right shit. Wolf, dog, fox, whatever. Even if the fake proverb is very 'Live, Laugh, Love', very 'Keep Calm and Carry On', it's what I need to hear right now.

I keep the proverb in mind and think about having a pet wolf.

*

The last time I was in this pub was for a wake. Now I feel awake. I'm fifteen minutes late. Just got to own it.

26

She's already teased me on text. I push open a large wooden door and she's the first person I see. Didn't have to look about or anything. Green eyes. Black leather jacket. The pub smells like a bass guitarist. Until she stands up to greet me. Her scent is fancy. She's tall. Softly spoken. We sit down.

Alternative education. Past lives. We're discussing all kinds of stuff. I order a whisky on the rocks and sip it slowly. She orders a glass of red. It all feels calm and medium. Nothing too extreme, just winding. We're sat by the bar and the stools are high. Tapped shoes for a second. She gets up to nip to the toilet. I turn towards a wall of bottles and catch my own reflection in a gap between the fridges and the shelves. I feel calm. I know she's very pretty but I don't feel desperate. I'm not assuming anything. We could easily have these drinks and be friends. I certainly don't have to feel intimidated. I'm young and I have time and money. I have good friends. I go to the gym. I'm interested in everything. I'm proud of myself, if anything. All of this is supposed to happen.

She smokes. I love smoking. We're outside now. Just about squeezing onto one of the benches. Everyone here looks like a tortured genius. Former druggie. Raver turned property tycoon. Smoking's always been a space of refuge for me. A panic break. She's telling me about her modelling career. That she's really an actor. Difficult transition. Pretty prejudice. It's a real thing. Her childhood. My childhood. Quite soon perhaps, but we figure it's a good sign. We only touch on it, then travel elsewhere. Find ourselves in the belief of the beyond. Begin to notice similarities. Coincidences perhaps. Signs, if you're feeling frisky. I'm really into numerology at the moment. Life paths. I figure her number out. It's the same as mine. Eleven.*

We talk about the fact that both of us had other plans before that club night. But both decided to move them to see our favourite artist, Anderson .Paak. I didn't drink. She didn't drink much. Only met her because I knew her friend and her friend needed to be held. Nudged. Reminded not to fall all over me. She'd taken too much MDMA. The gig was so good though. Music is an important point of relation. It all feels rhythmic. There are differences. She says she loves jewellery. Shows me this diamond ring. I hate diamond rings. Diamonds aren't even rare. She explains that it's vintage, that the pleasure is in there being an external reminder of how much you value yourself. I hear that. She then takes me through her other pieces. Both of our mothers love crystals and have passed it on. Hippie heritage. A rare quartz. Citrine. She then gently slides one ring up her third finger and says it's her favourite. Labradorite. I can't help smiling. I rest my hand on the uppermost part of my chest so I can feel the wolf's face. I follow the shape of the string until it meets fresh air. Tuck my hand behind my stripy t-shirt. Pull out my necklace.

---

* Listen, mid-twenties this kind of mysticism was a common point of connection. Don't care now I'm older. Yes, it's a fuckboy strategy. Was I a fuckboy? Yes. That's why I'm writing this. Look up your life path though. It's fascinating. Do it and then tell me you're not even tempted to look up someone else's. Yes, pseudo mysticism can be used manipulatively. Feminist fuckboys.

6

Four Months and Three Weeks Before

Chloe and I are in a different pub now.

The last thing Chloe asked me on our first meeting was which track is my favourite on Kendrick Lamar's new album. I read that as exciting and cute. Waited two minutes before I texted her and she texted straight back. Something was telling me I deserve this. Having just come out of something heavy, in which I was not the best version of myself. It was on and off. My first love. Fractured. Consistent. Engulfing.

Things got tough with my ex, Suzy. She was the one I was with when I became famous. I'd just earned my first proper bit of money the first night I met her. She says her interest in me wasn't anything to do with that. I could afford to buy both of us drinks. That must have been a contributing factor.

We were a bunch of barely legal butterflies flapping their way through Brighton's Lanes. Closed shops. Mouths open. Damp pavement. She kissed me first, actually. Pushed me up against some shutters. It was kind of dramatic. I couldn't believe my luck. Her reputation had preceded her. Stories of her asking boys to cum on her tits. Incredibly desirable. Sought after. A real-life fantasy female. I pretended I didn't know who she was when we first met. But she knew I knew. She had all the power then. Most of the stares between us in those initial meetings felt like I was being sized up. Evaluated. Deciding whether or not she could be bothered to blow my mind. I felt like I was one step away from being teased. One shifty response from exile. Once she'd decided that she wanted me, that was it. We had sex that first night. I can't remember it. Might have been shit. From then on it was tingly stomachs and tennis texting. And I could afford the hotel rooms and room service. Free breakfast.

We decided to make it official on the stroke of midnight one New Year's Eve. All I can remember is ordering a Southern Comfort and lemonade then standing on a table. Balloons, noise. Three, two, one. Shall we be boyfriend and girlfriend? Yes. Hooray. Friends outside. Hooray. Totally fucked. Two bottles of WKD and a lollipop. Helps with the jaw-swing. Spent most of the night-slash-morning on my mate's sofa. Wandered back to mine before dawn. Sun's up, got a girlfriend. We made sure that we both remembered the agreement we'd made. Confirming the commitment. We were both happy. At that time. She was renting a house in Deptford. Had a hot tub. Long story. Actually, it's not. Tragic loss lead to inheritance. Decided to enjoy it. Tattoo and a treasured ring. Which she gave to me. Quite soon into us being in a relationship she took the ring off her finger and slipped it onto my necklace. A fucking leap of faith. A solid-gold admission of trust.

*

We're actually about to leave this pub, Chloe and me. We decided to meet here last minute before I disappeared for a month for a TV show. Schedules had to be moved. We had to stick our thumbs into the glue. Didn't want it drying up. So we came here to talk more and feel each other out more and just make sure and look at each other's faces and analyse them and be cute and not rush and be blind to everything but in an adorable way. We smoke outside again, knowing that we're parting ways. Hands in pockets, hips swinging side to side. You know the one. Unsure what to do. She says she's cold so I offer her my fleece. Very chivalrous, although the thought of that makes me gag a bit. Her cab pulls up so I improvise a gesture so concrete it would set my footprint. I take my wolf necklace from around my neck and place it around hers. She asks me if I'm sure and I say yeah. Of course. Protect it. She smiles and jumps in the car. Door shut. Feeling weightless.

We named the wolf Alice.

7

Two Weeks *After* It Happened

The body never lies, does it. It contorts, opens, closes, wraps itself round itself. Tells stories our mouths can't. Argues with our expressions. Gives the game away sometimes. Yells clues. I've always been fascinated. Watched videos on it. My mum tells me everything's fine but the skin around her thumbs says different. Her chipped nail varnish. I've only got one light on in the living room. I'm underneath it. A gentle interrogation. For a couple of weeks now I've carried a dead animal. On my shoulders. I've had a dead carcass on my back. Maybe it's not even dead. Just feels like it is. I've made that assumption from the weight. I'm aching. From the guilt.

My mum's living here at the moment. Short on money. I'm trying to help her out. I've given her my flat and moved to Margate. It's October. Barely evening but dark already. Not my favourite time of year. Even if the autumn leaves remind me of my grandma. Mainly been at my girlfriend's in London. Hard to escape. First thing my mum did was put plants on the balcony. And little fairy lights. Brought it to life. Immediate maternal energy. Prior to her moving in, that balcony was 70 per cent pigeon shit. I'd attempted to let pigeons live there. As an act of kindness. As if they'd return it. Hoping they'd finish building the nest, then start on a Portaloo. I'm a wishful thinker.

The offering of my flat was intended as a repayment. I've always felt indebted to my mum for giving birth to me. Made it my life mission to give her everything I possibly could. I figured you couldn't do more than give someone a place to live. Even if it's come at my expense. Even if it's shifted me out of the city. She's smoking a cigarette at the dinner table. Ashing into a frosted glass tray laden with scarlet-tainted butts. She's always hated non-stick lipstick. I suppose I'm here looking for some rope. Or an umbilical cord. Hoping she'll say something wise and definitive. Like she often does. Near impossible, seeing as I haven't even told her what's going on. I've got another bomb in my gut.

She's trying to engage with me but the ticking is loud. It's reverberating off my silence. I try to cover the echoes with monosyllabic replies. Breathing life into the facade. I know she's complaining about something. Sometimes I think that if there was nothing to fight against, my mum would just disappear. Like in *Star Trek*. The world needs people like her though. People who care too much.

'Are you alright, honey?'

No, I'm not alright. I say that I am and apologise. A modern human impulse. But I can feel the lack of illumination. I agree with my mum about overhead lights. They're too much. I don't want a home to feel like a shop. But I'm not sure I can see anything. I know that somewhere in front of me is a big flat-screen television. Stuck to the wall. A hung abyss of scheduled horror. Just beneath it is a long white storage unit. A home mainly to dead games consoles and irrelevant DVD boxsets. The Ultimate Bond collection. Ultimately untouched and dusty. To the right of that, the wall has a slight partition. Separating this room from the kitchen. It's wide enough for me to have stuck a bunch of Polaroids on with Blu Tack. Forever memories of heady junctions. Most of the pictures document intimate, drug-fuelled nights. Behind me is an incredible print by a graphic designer friend of mine called Ziggy. He used to be sober. I watched him relapse on the kitchen counter just along from the partition. Didn't sleep for two days.

I can't see any of it. I'm in a one-horse race. Ticking, galloping. It's all merging into a single sound. I do that thing when you ask someone a question but don't want the answer. Cryptically search for confirmation.

It's always better to be honest, right? Next question.

Your partner should know every part of you, right?

My mum uses this African drum as a table. It's got a smell about it. Like sweet, earthy straw. Been in my life for years. All of my life. It's comforting. There's always a little bit of ash to brush off its skin. Right now its skin's partially bathed by the same lamp as me. On it there's a small book. Just between a fruit bowl and another ashtray. Very small. Called *The Little Book of Happiness*. Also been in my life forever. I remember it being by the toilet in my old house. A bookshelf in another. Nestled between a couple of CDs back in Neasden. A simple, drawn sunset on the cover. Faded orange. Eastern-looking. A design you might see in a dojo. My mum is humming. I reach out my left hand and pick the book up. As I bring it back towards me, the motion throws the scent of old pages. I breathe in. Scan the cover. Think for a moment. Open it at random.

'Possession is the root of all unhappiness.'

Of all pages, it's this page. Sucker for a sign. This is a painful one. I don't like being possessed. I don't like being possessive. Pride myself on it. Don't get ownership. The more you have, the more there is to lose. And yet here I am. Holding on to a delusional reality. Because I've lied. I'm living in a reality that exists only because I'm trying to control it. Doesn't feel genuine. Feels fake. Out of sorts with who I am. The version of me that lives in here isn't real. The version of me that she knows and claims to love is fictitious. Mythical. A fabricated whisper. It's unbelievable.

In order for me to truly believe in this love, I have to face my actions. I've been in this situation too many times now. Every time, in fact. I have a twist. A sting. An opposition to my spritely disposition. A counterbalance to my exuberance. The outskirts of the spotlight. She could be the one to understand. Accept me at my worst. My weakest. But praise the honesty. See it as a signifier of promise.

I used to believe you shouldn't say anything. That it was selfish to. I'd say that guilt was the price you pay. And a reminder that you care. That's the punishment. But in my experience, the energy seeps out in other ways. Lies actually require energy to maintain. And the fear's like a yappy dog. Running forwards, looking back.

Something's got to give. It wasn't so long ago that I googled 'can you be in love and depressed at the same time?' This could be a doorway. Everything you want is on the other side of fear. I am definitely most scared about being honest about what I've done. I'm confident that I want to be with this woman for the rest of my life. If she can hold me after I do this, I will be certain. I shut the book, look my mum dead in the eyes and tell her that I'm going. She adjusts immediately. Sits back in her chair. She will always make room for determination. I leave the flat. Step out into the crisp, smoky air. Hands in pockets. Striding into autopilot.

This feeling of holding on, I've had it before. I remember holding on when I first smoked DMT. Literally held on for dear life. DMT is the chemical that your brain emits when you dream and when you die. Comes out of the pineal gland. It also exists naturally. You can find it, smoke it and leave the planet – if you do it right. I smoked it with a man called Rob who lives on an estate in Archway. He's predominantly a part-time actor and deep tissue masseuse. Interdimensional travel is his hobby. Says he felt an obligation to share the experience. He's tall, smiley, calm, and has a fluffy cat. Spoke of a girlfriend I never met. Walked me into a room at the back of the flat. Had a whole relaxing place set up. Massage table pushed to the side. Lights off, blinds shut. Started with deep breathing. Stuck on music to aid the journey. My heart was fucking pounding. Three sharp inhalations. Hold my breath. Count to thirty. Rob said the plan is to cycle that process three or four times. My last memory was him getting to the number eight. Then I died.

Nothing could have prepared me for what I experienced. The last breath I pushed out was a consequence of my spirit having gone somewhere else. I wasn't in control of that breath. I couldn't feel any part of my body. If anything, I could feel spots of energy around it. Kaleidoscopic, intense, rich, unreal colours and shapes. Hues more defined than anything I'd ever seen in my life. The highest definition you could imagine. It was magical and terrifying. After a few minutes I began to worry about my body a little. I could hear my thoughts. I opened my eyes very briefly. Rob's hands were hovering over my chest. Attempting to centre my energy. My heart was beating really fucking fast. I travelled in between states for a few more minutes before settling in my body again completely. Opened my eyes. Burst out giggling.

Cosmic giggle, Rob called it. A natural reaction to the discovery that life in and of itself is a bit of a joke. The body giggles, having visited another dimension where none of this shit matters. Having felt and seen stuff unavailable on earth. Words can't describe it. They're limited. Rob told me the whole experience was about seven or eight minutes in total. Asked me what I saw and felt. I relayed as best I could. He said that I was fighting to stay in my body. Said the trip can be longer if I allow it to be. Offered another few tokes, given that I went under so quickly. Encouraged me to take deeper inhalations.

I inhaled again. Left my body. Freaked out. Came back into my body. Similar experience. Still trippy. Don't think I can do much more. The smell and taste of the DMT was so ruthless. As if its smoke was from a yelling throat. Powerful shit. Scary, law-defying shit. I left his flat feeling tuned in. Over the following week or so, whenever I thought about my experience or shared it, I'd feel this tiny, irritating void. A cylinder of absence. I hadn't quite done something. I suspected it was to do with the trip. I was off-kilter.

I messaged Rob and asked if I could book another trip.

He agreed. A week later I'm back in the room. DMT rolled up in my fingers, Rob with the lighter at the ready. Figured I'd already done this, didn't have to be so scared. I know what it feels like to leave my body. I can focus on the experience, not the shock. Took three sharp tokes. Counted to thirty. Got to about eleven. I was gone. Absolutely freaked out. Came back into my body at the same time as the other trips. More off kilter. I decide it's too much. I tell Rob I'm done and start getting my shit together. Rob stops me and says, 'Listen, I'm not going to force you to do anything that you don't want to do. But I feel obliged to suggest you try smoking it one more time. You need to stop fighting it and surrender. Completely let go of the experience. It's like swimming. The more you struggle, the harder it is.'

It wasn't his intention but I felt challenged. He might as well have said 'I double dare you'. I had to give it one more go. My expectations were low. Last try. Might as well inhale as much as possible and fucking go for it. Three sharp inhalations. These ones are deeper. I can't remember which number I got to. But in no time at all, I was gone.

After about five minutes, a thought appeared.

This is usually when I go back into my body.

That was the thought. Except this time it was separate to me. Somehow I was outside it. I don't know where I was. But I was aware that the thought was happening. Instead of experiencing it. That's when I knew. I was out. Completely. I had stepped outside my conscious mind. It sounds made up, but I promise this happened. A portal appeared. That's the most apt word I can find for what I saw. It had letters around it. I can't remember what they were. Maybe they weren't letters. I went through it. And I was no longer me.

I wasn't a person. With fears and dreams and questions. There was no 'I'. It's difficult to explain. There was no past, present or future. I swear time didn't even exist where I was. It wasn't a unit of measurement. I was just drifting through an expansive, eternal bed of turquoise. And I felt myself being guided through by a distinctly womanly energy. Or maternal? I don't know. I couldn't see or understand what or who the energy was but I could feel it. Feel her. I saw mechanical butterflies. Felt as though I was cumming. Infinitely. As though I'd exploded and all that remained was pleasure. Sensuality. Pure, uncut bliss. Forever. Blue-green ecstasy. Bursting where the land meets the sea.

I opened my eyes. My jaw had dropped and my palms were facing the sky. I had repositioned while elsewhere. As though I'd been practising meditation since I was born. Felt like I'd just been to where I was before I was born. I accepted the fact that I was back and literally jumped up from where I'd been sitting. Like a springboard. Fucking alive. Clutching my face like 'The Scream' painting. Laughing inside. Laughing outside. Rob starts nodding. He's beaming too.

'You saw it, didn't you?' he said. 'You went there.'

*

I just need to let go. Right now that's my only choice. I'm halfway to Chloe's. It's only a fifteen-minute walk. She has said it's important for partners to live near each other. I argued that living in the same city is enough. Either way I'm walking into this. It's just me, the gaps between the pavement and the trees. I haven't even seen another person this whole time. I'm in a slipstream. On a ride at a terrifying water park. Water is terrifying if you think about it. It knows no bounds. Best thing to be though. Water.

I arrive at her door. Autopilot still in full effect. So many voices. Questioning. Challenging. Fear. Don't do it. It'll be fine. Nothing to worry about. You're underestimating her. She loves you. She'll forgive you. I put the key in. Walk in. She's in the middle of something. Folding clothes. Quick hello. Nice to see me. Very usual. I'm heavy. I walk straight into the kitchen. That's where we usually talk. Eventually she walks in. Pulls up at the sight of my brows probably. The angle of my head. Dog took a shit on the bed kind of look.

'Are you alright?' she says.

It's been two weeks. I left it two weeks to say something. A fortnight of conflict. Most people told me not to say anything. But it was coming out regardless. In my choice of words. Irritability. Distance. I'd pray for a soft entry. A lifeline. Perhaps she'd adapted her view on partnership. On commitment and monogamy. I'd prod cryptically, relentlessly, hoping she'd lost faith in tradition. Or become open to non-conventional approaches. Of course she hadn't. Her boundaries were firmly in place. Straightforward agreements. Black and white. And here I am in hellish grey. Casting shade. Abusing the tone. There's a chance that she would have never found out. But that space was uninhabitable. Our connection was based on a dead idea of who I am.

'I have to tell you something,' I say. Leaning against the

kitchen countertop. Her directly in front. One leg cocked up against the radiator. Doesn't feel like it's on. That sentence was a starting pistol. I half hope I fall into the oven. I can't feel my legs. I can't feel the words leave my mouth. They snake between us. I pretend I'm not bleeding.

'What?' she replies.

All my non-verbal cues are deafening.

'I hooked up with someone else.'

Below zero. Bright red. Her hair seems thicker. Electric. I'm drawn to everything about her that I find attractive. Cruel mind. She asks when. I say at the wedding. She says that was two weeks ago. I say I know. Now there's silence. I start fizzing. I can't hold it together. A reserve tank kicks in. An army of defensive thoughts rocket into my imagination. Create a fort. Rapidly summarise why I've got nothing to be afraid of. I simply have to get my point across. It's just a case of me explaining why this isn't as bad as it sounds.

She asks what happened.

I'm answering honestly. This must be the right thing to do. It feels transactional but might be less so once it settles.

'I was completely out of it. I took a shit-tonne of drugs and fucked up. I wasn't in a good place but I'm going to deal with it.'

I'm nothing. My emotion somewhere out of the window. Lodged in my past. I feel so far from crying. Tears would be useful right now. To show that I care. I really fucking care but I can't show it. I'm just blank. Answering questions. Like a statue. I've barely moved.

There are cracks beneath me.

'You have to understand it's got nothing to do with you.

I wasn't trying to hurt you. I was hurting myself. Honestly. I'm sorry.'

Of course it's got something to do with her.

'It's not personal. I don't know how to explain it. I didn't want it to happen. Please believe me. I fucked up. I know I did . . .'

She's calculating everything. Emotionally. Balancing scales I've leapt over. I hadn't thought of any of this. Hadn't pre-empted these crossroads. I'd just felt something and made a decision. Now I feel like a fridge freezer. Tipped precariously. A bunch of eggs rolling freely inside.

'Please. You have to believe me. This is my problem . . .'

It is my problem. I have a real issue with self-destructing. A dark, repetitive cycle. Drug abuse. Fleeting validation. Sex. Control. Love. These are all my issues. I had them before her and they've got me round the fucking throat. I make it clear that I'm telling her because I want things to be different. It's an indication that I want to change. And I have enough belief in our love to be truthful. It's taken me two weeks to tell her because it wasn't an easy decision. But I've still waited to tell the truth. And this whole time I knew. I hadn't planned on cheating. I'm hoping she just needs some more time to think about it. All other sides of me are great. Surely that's enough. I'll just continue leaning here. All weight on my shoulders. Tight, tense muscles. Clenched neck. Holding position. I breathe in the faint scent of her cat's litter tray. Notice the magnets on the fridge. The cork board to the left of her. The pinned photograph of her wearing the wolf necklace at an event. It can't all disappear.

I just need Chloe to understand. I need her to understand

that if she forgives me in this moment I would never ever do it again. Sometimes you don't realise what you have until you've risked losing it. I know now how much she means to me. As people always say, too little, too late.

I told Chloe that I loved her incredibly quickly. I was overcome with it. Felt it early. And even before those words were exchanged I'd say, 'I believe you.' At the end of messages. And the end of notes. I'd write bits and show her in the hope she'd do the same. One of the early pieces I wrote was about a holiday I went on as a kid. Package holiday. Affordable. Ridiculous. There was a beach though. And it was hot. A miracle for a mother and son living on an estate. I remember leaving her side and walking into the ocean. I must have been about 10. I headed into the big blue and let the waves hug me. They felt friendly. But it was only a few steps between me being knee-deep and up to my shoulders. I turned around to face my mum. Big smile. Like I'd stuck an orange peel in there. She smiled orange back. Seeing her son in the ocean bouncing like a ray of sun on the ocean. Then I felt a wave knock the back of my head. I winced. Ocean briefly covered my mouth. I tried not to swallow. Funny how something so soft can become so scary. I wasn't happy any more. Wasn't enjoying myself. My mum could see it. Reacted instantly. The soles of her feet hit the sand hard. She was wearing a sarong. Clutched it as she paced over with her free arm outstretched. That's the first time I felt like I was drowning.

'Get out of my house,' Chloe says, 'Get out.' 'Please,' I say. 'Can we just talk?' 'No. Get out.' It's a cigarette-in-mouth situation. I can feel my chest suddenly. It's tight.

Like a scared old woman with a purse. Heartbeat off the scale. Shifting scales. It can't all disappear.

'Let me just explain myself,' I say. 'Please, Chloe. I'm begging you.'

'Leave my house,' she says. I'm stiff. Rusty. Lost. I'm hesitant to turn my back to the kitchen but I have to. I have to head down this hallway. Past the framed flowers. Along the wooden floorboards. Along those planks. Out into the fresh emptiness of the evening. Into an ocean of messy circles. Unfinished shapes.

It's only once I'm outside that I defrost. A layer melts. The air is sharp. This street's hidden. But right now it feels detached. Broken away entirely from reality. Somewhere across that void is a normal London where no one makes mistakes. There is a break. Inside me I feel a break. My insides are in pain. The pain crawls up the back of my throat. Dislodges a rock. That rock falls down onto my chest. Starts an avalanche. And my airway is clear. My eyes start streaming. My belly retracting like it's firing a water pistol. Everything is crying now. I'm sobbing. I can't go home. I'm in pieces. The dam is done.

I get my phone out and ring Tai.

8

A Young Father

'Jesus loves pussy!'

I met a guy once who said that to me in the gym. Big South African dude. Six six and butch. Could've been in *Game of Thrones*. Laughed like a hyena. He was being openly homophobic. In spite of a healthy number of the gym members being gay. Including close friends of his. Made no sense. Felt like an act. His gay mates probably thought it was an overcompensation. I asked him if he was religious. He said that he obviously was. Like I was supposed to know. So I asked him why God put the male G-spot up the arse. His face froze. Wheel of death on his forehead. Couldn't compute. I carried on. Attempting to remain impartial. Further making the point. If God created everything, then why did he put it there? The ultimate orgasm. Right up our arses. I suggest that it's some kind of cruel joke. Odd though, all the same. Animals are gay too, I reminded him. I bet he's seen a few dogs try and fuck each other.

His brain did a force quit. Ignored most of my points. Jumped to a place of safety. No word of a lie. Exclaimed 'Jesus loves pussy!' while jumping around. Like a child after a chocolate bar. Repeated it until conclusion. I'd already had my fun. I let him cartwheel.

The gym is a zoo. And at this gym a few members did go purely to observe. They called them cruisers. Old gay dudes looking for fresh meat. Quite unsettling. When I first started going, this guy used to just stare at me. Sometimes in the mirror, sometimes not. Didn't even put a pin in the stacks he was lifting. Not even an attempt to hide it. Stood there flapping his arms up and down like a failed demolition. Hoping for an explosion.

I started going to the gym because a friend called me fat. While we were on holiday. All the boys I went on holiday with were fucking skinny. I posed for a photo and he said I looked like a 'beached whale'. I hadn't been aware of my body until then, really. I'd just been eating everything I wanted to eat. Had no mum to cook for me any more. I was just young, rich, famous and loved apple pie for breakfast. Tai was suggested to me when I enquired about working out.

When he told me that apple pie was unhealthy it blew my mind. That was the extent of my knowledge at that point. Hot cross buns too. Fucking devastated.

Gym became a new addiction. I loved seeing Tai and I loved getting into shape. The rush of endorphins. I had abs and I felt strong. I started eating these tailor-made meals. Meals that guaranteed muscle growth. I'd get compliments on my new physique. I bathed in them. Became attached to them. Looked forward to taking my top off. At one point I was cycling everywhere, playing football twice a week, going to the gym three times a week and doing yoga. I found it difficult to stop. Then I got injured. I fucked up my wrist and my ankle within three days. Meaning I couldn't train at all. At that point I had been eating four or five meals a day. Suddenly I was doing fuck all but with a huge stomach. I kept eating but began to panic that I wouldn't be able to lose the weight again. That I'd return to physical mediocrity. No smirk when the shirt's lifted. I started clutching at parts of my body to see if they felt fatty. Mostly my stomach. It became so obsessive that even since regaining my shape, I will clutch at my body whenever I'm anxious. It's just part of that neural pathway. My desperation to have no fat on me flares up dependent on how I'm doing in life. Honestly, I think it's become dysmorphia.

Tai's not far off it either. The way we talk to each other about our bodies is probably quite unhealthy but it's one of our bonds. One of many. I don't think we expected to become so close. A trainer–trainee relationship can be transactional. And yet we intertwined. I worked hard. I loved talking. He started off telling me to shut up and do my set. Ended up engaging in existential debates for most of the session and feeling guilty he'd charged me. Seems I'd filled an intellectual chasm in his life. He's obsessed with learning. Finding out new information. He loves it. He's fucking bright.

He's a young father. Had a child in his early twenties. Raises that child pretty much on his own. Beautiful boy. Jules. Must be wonderful having a dad so loving. Nurturing. His remaining paternal energy is spent on his ex-girlfriend.

And the whole time he was raising this beautiful young boy. Who has a smile like parting clouds. And he would emphasise how important it was for him to have consistent figures in his life. For his development. Especially boys like older brothers. Tai could never have had another child with Jules's mum. He is an emotionally driven, love-orientated man. But romantic choices aren't his strong suit.

I ring Tai and ask to come over. He says yes. I am sobbing after all. Crying really clicks people into gear. If it's authentic, it's undeniable. It's human to move towards it. Part of me wishes I'd cried back at Chloe's. There are so many times in my life that I could have done with tears. I'm walking up to Tai's, streaming. Darkness, wind and tears. I'm gliding there miserably. Lost track of time completely. Heart's going through the roof. I get to Tai's, knock on the door and burst in. Three flights of stairs. Plain white walls. Undecorated but homely. A few toys and gadgets scattered about. Comfy communal area in the open-plan living room. That's where we'd smoke weed and watch dumb shit. A hundred chocolates and *The Walking Dead*. A womb of sorts. He's done the maths by this point. He figures I must have told her.

He told me not to tell her when I asked him if I should. Two weeks ago. He said she wouldn't react well. He's also been cheated on. So he concluded I keep quiet. I turned up here in a similar fashion a day after it happened. He was having a party. Four to the floor, jaws swinging. I'd drunk a little but not much. I felt too tight. Wasn't moving fluidly at all. All I could think about was what I'd done and what I should do about it. Still in shock. And you never know how it's going to feel, you just have to guess. Like dropping an iPhone. You do your best to avoid it. But when it happens all you can think about is getting the screen fixed. Survival mode. Tai told me I shouldn't say anything and I ignored him. I was eating myself alive, couldn't handle it. And even that night. I remember meeting some other friends down by the canal. Drinking by a houseboat. And there was a new woman there. Friend of a friend. And she was staring at me. A lot. And it made my stomach feel funny. My sick stomach. Still felt excited somehow. The validation was intoxicating. And it felt so rare that a woman looked at me like that. Genuinely. It would enter my mind that I would never have that moment again. Right now an attractive woman is actually asking me to fuck her. That must be what that stare meant. Head slightly tilted. You know the one. Dilated pupils. Little grin. Lust blots. Like water on paper. There's a whole story there. How can I not read it? Even with this guilt sat in my stomach like hot tar, I still fantasise. And have to pull myself away. Because that validation feels so rare to me. To me as a man. We're the ones who stare. I felt like a poster boy. Let me make those dreams come true. Fuck the consequences. I've grown up taking opportunities. That's how I am where I am. But I left. And then thought about it for days. Probably wanked over it.

He asked me why I told her and I lay a tube map. Perfectly measured trains of thought that result in a fault-less destination. I rationalise it, break it down, say I told her because I figured it was a step forwards. I was opening a window. Couldn't stand how stuffy it was in my head. A space heated by regret. I used to think that was what you had to do. Sweat it out. But I wanted to face the fresh air. It wasn't supposed to sting this much. I convince myself that it makes sense to forgive me. It's irrational not to, surely. Tai suggests that cheating on someone doesn't encourage rationality. I can't control another person's reaction. I text her and ask if we can speak about it. She quickly replies no. I always manage to figure things out. I can't imagine this ending in a sum I can't balance. I have no idea how I'm going to sleep. Tai lets me smoke inside. His son is staying at his mum's. Thank God. Doesn't have to see me like this. Choking. Eyes stinging. Red throat. Uncut panic. Barren cave of a mouth. Bats disturbed by the fumes. I lie down on the sofa. That's where I'm going to sleep. Tai sits at his dinner table, drinks a glass of water. Asks me if I need something to help myself go unconscious. Says I've got to get through to the morning. Reproach the terror with aid from the sun. If there is any sun. It's almost November. Seventy per cent rain in England. I wonder if that contributes to the self-destruction. Sleeping pills are an option. A spliff. I go for the spliff. Feels less intense. Bound to make things lighter. Ease the pain. Past laughter nudges my thumb. I spark the lighter hoping for relief. Take a hard toke. Tai warmly bows out, goes to get some sleep. I stare at the ceiling as my thoughts snake.

I'm a lightweight smoker. Smoked my first spliff at around 12 years old. Sucked in dramatically and held my breath for a stupid amount of time. Never been able to function properly when stoned. All I think about is food and sleep. And the in-between thoughts I have are more reflective of the dissociative space I find myself in. Concerned voices. Only there because I'm stoned, but concerned that I'm stoned. Lateral murmurs. My basic perception morphs into a myriad of questions. Sat at one end of the stick. And the entire world is at the other end. Tai actually says that he loves me getting stoned because

I become a moron. He says he relates more to me then 'cause I'm at his level. Food does taste phenomenal. In a comfortable setting it's still a great pastime.

I don't think anywhere would be comfortable for me right now. My legs are too long for the sofa. I'm planning to get into the foetal position soon, so it doesn't matter. The ceiling feels like it's lowering. I can feel the smoggy hug of the spliff in my system. But once it's in my brain, it isn't fun. It's not fun and it's not comforting. I start to think about every possible outcome of this scenario that leaves me looking awful. Every exit leading to a sheer drop. I crawl towards states of being where I can pretend this night isn't happening at all. And feel relief for a few moments. But then I remember that it is very real. It feels even worse. What goes up must come down. And I'm high. And in another sense I've been high for a long time. Coasting. Getting my own way. Drifting over walls other people are busy climbing. Smirking to myself. There's no way over this wall right now. Solid brick heading straight into the heavens. I head-butt it till I'm unconscious.

I've got nothing to say to you. Come and get your stuff.

9

The Mourning After

Morning. Tai assures me that she'll find forgiveness. The day is clear. My mind isn't. Barely slept. I plead via text. She's not having any of it. I wonder if it's too early to smoke. I decide not to take my ADHD pills. The ones I've been self-medicating with. Maybe they're at the root of all this. Haven't been myself. Bizarrely, I'd agreed to see a spiritual therapist today. Somebody I'd been connected to a while back through a woman I met on an app who gave me a sound bath. The woman is called Jessica and she is on another level. Literally. Speaks to spirits. These kinds of people often appear in my life. Likely a continuation of my mum's belief in heightened states. Alternate realities. Ancient energies. My mum has always encouraged me to give thanks to my allies and ancestors. Had me doing Native American card rituals. Burying crystals. Reminds me of the amethyst I had next to my crib as a baby. Says it gave me powers.

First time I had a session with Jessica, she came over to my flat. Before I handed it over to my mum. Asked me if I'd ever done any spirit work before. I said yeah, with my mum etc. Then she said that on the way over to mine she kept having visions of Atlas. As in the mythological Greek dude carrying the world on his back. Claimed the image appeared to her in preparation for seeing me. Said I was carrying a similar weight on my shoulders. Still fucking am.

Right now is not the best time. I text Jessica and tell her that I'm in the middle of an awful breakup. Maybe we should reschedule. She texts back and suggests we go ahead. Claims the timing couldn't be better. I ask Tai if he'd be ok with her coming here. He agrees while making us breakfast. That beautiful, nurturing energy. Eggs and porridge. I eat what I can. He makes a double espresso and heads off to the gym. As much as he wants to stay he can't let his clients down. I didn't expect him to stay. He's very loyal and doesn't like to cancel plans. Probably good that Jessica is coming here. I don't want to be left by myself. The front door shuts and I wiggle my toes. I realise I haven't felt them for a long time. Years. Where have my toes been this whole time? I've been walking on them. But they must have lost their nerve. Bloodless. My therapist did suggest I'd been living from the neck up. Detached from my torso like a piece of Lego. Child's play. Out of body. Head in the clouds. I can feel my gut though. That's never gone.

A couple of hours later Jessica arrives. Short, frantic, strawberry blonde, smelling of roll-ups. Proper London accent. Essex even. That twang. She looks a little apprehensive. Probably 'cause I look a little apprehensive. Quite an intense meeting. Dealing with someone whose heart has snapped in half. She sits on one of the two sofas. Takes a deep breath, assesses the space a bit, asks me what happened. I launch into a tirade, pleading my innocence. Leaving it beyond doubt. Jessica squints a little. Like I'm a boat on the horizon.

'But . . . I don't understand . . . how do you expect her to react?'

This is how. Everything would go as it went, except instead of ordering me to get out, she pauses. Thinks for a long time. Looks up at me. Looks me dead in the eyes. Acknowledges my regret.

Reads it. Asks me why I got so fucked up. Understands it as a relapse. Balances that reality with her own fury. Doesn't kick me out. Says she needs time but understands I didn't mean to hurt her. Calls me an idiot. Something like that. But ultimately sees the situation for what it is. Sees me for who I really am!*

I say all this to Jessica really quickly. The more I talk, the more her eyes widen. Eventually both her eyebrows raise and she interrupts me.

'Ok. You need to slow down.'

I carry on protesting. Proving her point.

'Seriously. Stop.'

She holds one hand up. The other hand she has placed on a box she's pulled out of her bag while I was talking. She closes her eyes.

'I just need to tune in a second.'

I bite my tongue. Swallow it. Choke on it. I don't know what to do with the silence. Feels radioactive.

After a moment, she opens her eyes again. 'I need you to close your eyes.'

I don't respond.

---

* denial

'I need you to close your eyes and look for the little you.'

I attempt to compose myself and do what she says. I close my eyes. And I see myself instantly. The young me. The little, tiny me. Straight away. It's unbelievable. Vivid. Like I'm tripping. I don't know why, in this moment, I'm able to see. But I am. And it's really painful. I know exactly where I am. I'm in the living room where Mum and I used to live. Just down the road from where I am now. Kensal Rise. Keslake Road. Daytime. Sun hugging the room. Pressing its way through a pair of curtains. I'm facing them. The sofa is on the left. Covered by a throw with black and white patterns. One of the many we had. A quilt just next to it. Little me is sat in the centre of the room. Alone. Playing with an abacus. Chubby little legs in front. Hair full of ringlets. One side flat from where I'd been lying down. I'm in a nappy. Little me knows I'm there too. Looks up at me.

Hamster cheeks. You could see them from behind me. Hiding chestnuts and plans for the future. I'm open again. Eyes streaming. Warm rivers. A different kind of grief, this one. I'm reminded that this is a vision when I hear the faint patter of a tear drip onto Tai's sofa. Then I hear Jessica's voice.

'Can you see him?'

'Yes.'

'Ok.'

'Why haven't I seen him before?!' My eyes are still closed. I'm devastated.

'Don't worry about that right now, ok? Let's just stay calm and focused.'

'But what the fuck? It's so clear. It's like he's been here this whole time and I've just been ignoring him?'

'Ask him what he wants.'

I do. And the response is clear and honest. Short and sweet. Comfort. That's all he wants. Comfort. And I imagine all the times I've ignored him. All the times I've been unaware of needing him. Or the times when he has spoken and I've let it tumble away like a loose coin, spin to a standstill. I think he comes through when I'm writing. But I think of the creations as separate to myself. I wrote a song recently about intimacy issues, then thought 'that's cool' and carried on with my life. And now I'm realising. He's always tried to guide me in simple ways. With his simple emotions. And simple understandings. A simplicity I find terrifying. I've learned to make beds in blizzards. Backstroke into whirlpools. Moonwalk through lava. I welcome chaos. But this little me just feels. He holds bricks. That's it. Same shape, same weight. Just need to be held together.

I wonder if he tried to communicate to me when I jumped into black cabs. With grams of coke, dead phones and stale hope. Stale like the smell of piss outside the club. Trying desperately to follow a group of total strangers to a moderately famous person's house. Just to do more drugs. And entertain empty possibilities.

I don't have many memories of this first house in Keslake Road. Not solid ones. A thunderstorm comes to mind. The shock and excitement. Zigzags in the sky. Me and my cousin pegging it down the corridor to get to the back garden. Mum stood by the door, smiling. I couldn't see the sky, it was raining so much. But I wanted all the thunder. All the lightning. I couldn't believe the sky could do that. Still can't. Electrics in the sky. And my cousin. Sometimes. Would pack up a bunch of my toys in a tiny suitcase and march triumphantly out the house. As if that was an option. And those toys belonged to her. The suitcase was hers, to be fair. And actually those toys weren't 'mine'. We didn't believe in that growing up. My mum banned me from saying that word.

There's a gorgeous photograph of that living room. Of me and my cousin. And my gran.

My gran.

My gran.

My grandmother.

My dad's mum who died two years ago.

Comfort.

At her funeral, I said a few words. Was proud of them. Delivered them well. Smiled, sat down. Saw my mum welling up. I haven't been to many funerals but they've all been similar. Graveyard. Flowers thrown. Sunglasses. Black, black, black. Church-looking room. Religious guy saying things. Casket. Photos. My dad was sat across from us with his girlfriend. Head fallen into his chest. His long dreads concealing his face but his shoulders gave it away. He cried with his whole body. During the service in the graveyard he actually couldn't stand. His legs kept giving away under him. Knees shaking. I'd never seen my dad like that before. I think even he was shocked. But the whole time I remained poised. Told myself this was inevitable. She was almost 90 years old. She was bedridden. Could barely see. What else was going to happen? Yeah, it was sad, sure. But that's life, isn't it? Old people die. Entropy.

I didn't shed a single tear. For the woman who provided me with the only space I truly felt safe as a child. A space I felt comfortable. And little me misses her. He misses her so much. And he has done, for years. He was shaking at that funeral.

Let me tell you. My gran lived halfway up a hill in Finchley. Split mansion. Four separate flats but looked grand from the outside. Been there forever. Since Windrush. You walk in the front but I preferred the fire escape. Same as the council estate I lived on. Feel the gaps in the grille as you climb them. Slide down the side of the building to get there. Check the garden as you go. The back garden. With the apple tree and winding patio. My gran would pick those apples and make stew. Warm apple stew with vanilla ice cream. Yeah, all of that. She'd let me dip strawberries in brown sugar. Serve up a bowl of whole milk and banana. Grandmother grandeur. But the garden was my favourite. I'd cartwheel, play football, float. While she sat, still. Grinning. Eyes closed sometimes. Her face was so full. All features plump with knowledge. Half-grey afro. I can only remember her getting sharp with me once. Everything else was patience and times tables. John Agard and *Chicken Soup for the Soul*. Poetry and numbers. We weren't always picking apples of course. That's a seasonal thing. My grandmother was a seasonal woman. She was autumn.

Hugging her was satisfying as crunching leaves. She was orange. Still warm when the world wasn't. You'd walk up the fire escape and into the main mansion-looking building. There'd be two identical doors. I used to think the other one led to hell. Her neighbour was a lifelong friend actually.

Paper stand by my gran's. Door open. Brushing wood over the carpet. Potpourri. The waft of dead flowers. Proper vintage. Kitchen just to the right. Bedroom to the right of that, but I never went in there. Not until she started to get ill. I was always straight down the corridor in front of the door. Into the main room. Collapsible dark wooden dining table. Two chairs. Fireplace. Two chairs. Dressing table with a fancy mirror. A bit regal. She was a bit regal. A big vase full of twigs. Bookcase full of books. A few old toy cars resting on the lesser-used shelves. Large sofa to the left. Large for me anyway. That's where I'd sleep. My grand-father's paintings hung above it. A grandfather I never met. They hung above the sofa, the television and the hi-fi. Didn't watch telly much, but the stereo was always on. Classic FM. She was obsessed. Could have been the key to her calm. Classical continuity.

My gran spent her final years in a home. Such a difficult part of existence. Such an odd smell. I would go straight to her room. Tried to go as much as possible with my mum and dad. He, of course, was there a lot. I was busy though. And I think I found it hard. Hard to watch a human being expire. Her body began to ache. She even-tually became too frail to carry herself. Became bedridden and could barely see. But she never forgot me. And even though she was often disorientated and a little confused, it wouldn't take much to make her smile. That orange beam. Sunset energy. And she sang. Right to the end. She didn't know the date, time or even where she was. But she would burst into songs she'd known for decades. Recite poems from her youth. They never left her. And after she'd passed I remember reading a letter written by a student of hers from her time as a teacher. Could have been thirty years before, maybe more. Sending their love and professing the effect that she'd had on them.

I hadn't felt this grief until now. Hadn't allowed myself to. Just swallowed it. But like I said, the dam's broken. Because of this breakup. This heart split. And I'm overcome with a true understanding of how important my grandmothers were to me. Another grief. I never met my grandfathers. They died before I was born. But my mum's mother too. I think of her and taste cinnamon. I see her pushing ingredients around a mixing bowl. Me salivating at the promise of rock cakes. She'd feed me elevenses. At that time I knew I'd be getting an assortment of nuts, raisins and a biscuit if I finished. Watching films with my cousins. Watching her do the crossword. Rarely being able to help her. I was the reason she got a hip replacement. First, because she once ran along beside me in the park while I was on a zip-wire tyre and was so fixated on my joy that she ran into a tree. The second time because I ran gleefully into her bedroom during one of my birthdays. Scared the shit out of her and she slipped on the skirting of her bed. Tried not to blame myself. Wondered if I was cursed. Dementia hit her a lot harder than my other gran. I'd go round to clean her windows and she began to get it in her head that I was stealing things. Accused me of trying to shift her stuff on *The Antiques Roadshow*. We used to watch that show a lot. She started to recite raunchy dreams to whoever was around. Moved around a lot. Ended up deciding that she wanted to die peacefully in a cottage further out from the city. In a place called Firle. Spooky place. Apparently one of the last places a witch was burned. Barely anyone there. One pub, one post office and an honesty box for vegetables. Too quiet for me as a kid turning teenager. It freaked me out that there weren't any sports shops. But I did like it. She had a neighbour called Clive who fixed watches and made jam.

The plan to die there didn't work. She ended up living for another eight years or something. Prolonged her life if anything. Eventually the dementia hit her so hard she too ended up in a home. An expensive one. Killed her life savings. Same as my dad's mum. So fucked up. And her response to the deterioration was different. She became a little nasty. Short with people. It upset my mum a lot. My mum was doing her best. She was never short with me, but there was an occasion when I visited her and she asked my mum who the 'handsome man' was. I guess my heart broke in that moment. But, again, I rationalised it. Felt like she'd already died. Struggled to understand why we were keeping her alive. Started writing stories about how much better it would be for everyone if I just killed her myself. I really felt as though that would have been the kindest thing to do. Perhaps I was dealing with the anger of grief. There's a chance it also made the most sense.

I loved the both of them. Deeply. And never dealt with it. So now I'm feeling it all at once. Amongst other things. It's all rising to the surface. Plastic balls pushed to the bottom of a pool. And my body is very much here. I know I have a body.

I open my eyes and Jessica knows. She has a good idea of what I'm experiencing. Especially as I hadn't until this point. She's gentle. Talks slowly. Hushed tones. She assures me that it's all part of a process. Right now I need to take care of myself. Which I'm sure I'll be hearing a lot. Gets me to breathe. Reminds me that we have each other's numbers. Says we can speak whenever. Makes alternate conversation. Not to distract but just to take the edge off. She herself is going through a lot – has gone through a lot. She's arrived at this point through battle. I feel that. And she cares a lot. She cares about people who are left to make houses with no tools. Like I say, she's tapped in. A medicine. She goes, and I continue to dwell. She suggested that I give Chloe some space. I agreed with her but now I'm going to text Chloe. She has to know what I've discovered.

10

Removal

Chloe says again that I need to come and get my stuff. I'm in shock. Totally open. Raw. Fucking vulnerable. I start writing her a letter. Getting my stuff means seeing her and seeing her means there's a chance she'll listen. I'm writing it all on my phone. I've got to find a way. With nearly everything in my life I've found a way to do things. To get what I want. Razor-sharp tongue. I've never felt so far from it but I've got to try. I have a career in writing words. Now is the time to tap into everything. I smoke cigarettes and write until Tai gets home.

I'm going sober. I'm coming off everything, including my ADHD medication. That's been hell anyway. I have no idea how much to take. Or how often. I got diagnosed when I was a kid and then again as an adult. Initially my mum kept me off medication, which I think was the right idea. But I was bouncing off the walls. I was briefly put into cognitive behavioural therapy at the local kids' mental health centre but I hated it. I remember sitting in a beige room in front of a white board and a man with glasses. He had longish hair tucked behind his ears. He looked like a bank heist computer hacker. He started drawing a

bunch of spider diagrams in an attempt to help me understand my brain. It felt quite condescending. I lost interest
quickly and he could tell. Eventually he gave up, stepped
towards me, looked around a little bit and asked if I had
ever tried 'smoking marijuana'. Said he'd heard that it
helps. Was probably trying to be on a level. I appreciated
the effort but never went back. Other than that I just got
put in a special room for my GCSEs with a load of dyslexic
kids and was told I could stand up whenever I wanted. If
I needed a piss, I was escorted to the disabled loos. Which
would have made cheating incredibly easy, given the added
space and lack of monitoring. I chose not to. Comfortably
missed all my target grades.

Ended up taking a form of medication not long after I'd
left college. Cocaine. Having not felt fully apprehended by
my ADHD at that point, I was unaware of the level of
focus I would achieve through stimulants. Often I would
do a line and shut the fuck up. Shocking, to be honest. I
would become fixated on things. Predictably, on nights out
those 'things' would be more drugs and sex. Or intense
conversations. Cocaine would also sober me up which
fueled a deepening destruction. I'd be known to drink so
much and take so much that I would pass out. Unlike some
of those around me I couldn't stay up for two days straight.
At a certain point my body would just switch off. I'd buzz,
then fuse. But it was all part of it. We were all getting
mashed up. Pure hedonism. And my experience wasn't
completely abnormal. I might not have snorted lines and
announced to rooms that I was Christ reincarnated but the
drugs definitely made me a lot more forward. And sharing
cocaine with women often hoovered into sex. Debauchery.

Adrenaline-fuelled fucking fuck it. Sex with women I wanted to have sex with and some I didn't. It was all part of the same high. A high founded on lows. A clear stream of questionless cloudy desire. Smoky lustful crossovers. Translucent souls trying to block out the daylight.

I loved cocaine because it quietened down the voices in my head. It stopped me questioning myself. Overthinking what people thought of me. It cushioned the chaos. Even if I had shit sleeps and made awful choices. I say this in the past tense because it also fucking ruined my life. Again. It's ruined my life and provided me with my greatest stories. My medals of dishonour. I worry life is nothing without it. But with it I can't seem to hold on to anything.

I first took cocaine on holiday when I was 17. We got it off a guy called Mr Cool. No lie. Not a joke either. I saw this guy turn up to a club and fall asleep on a sofa. We were getting into clubs with fake IDs. On this one night we were blagging to some girls that we were at uni. Blah blah. Decided to go off and give it a try. The cocaine, not uni. Two lines in the bog. Came back and drank seven mixers back to back. Like they were water. I was deep in conversation, just pouring more venom in the pot. At some point I said I was going to the toilet and ended up in the car park outside. Under a parked car. I'd been sick on myself twice. I came back round to see two girls looking down at me. Thought I might have been in heaven. Until I saw my friend part them and hold me up like a scene in a war movie. Once I fully regained consciousness I had a Red Bull and went back in.

The following years I began to get my head round it. And the thing about cocaine is it breeds heady escapes.

Just in the practicality of it. The chemistry. If there's someone you fancy and they fancy some cocaine then within moments you are there with the person you fancy often alone together in small rooms or toilets or whatever and then you snort the cocaine or fucking speed to be honest that's what's in it these days and then you get a rush of adrenaline pupils dilate start tonguing each other. Cocaine then sex all the time. Heart rate through the roof. Sometimes the sex would be on roofs. In parks. Fucking high as shit let's get it on. So frustrating when my brain got knocked though. Scratched memories. Some of the times I really wanted to remember in more detail. But it's patchy. Just vinegar vignettes. I suppose all the blood was running to different places. Sometimes I have no recollection of it at all. But cocaine mixed with the feeling of knowing you're about to have sex. Unreal. Addictive. Overwhelming. Character-altering. Madness.

So far this was hedonism. Chaos energy. Not yet a cocaine problem. The cocaine problem started on the nights when I didn't go out. I began to realise that the focus I was gaining from coke could be used productively. I'd buy a couple of grams. Sit there. Get fucking high. And write. I'd write so much. I'd get so much done. Hyper-productive. And I'd tell everyone. With such tenacity that it didn't seem like a problem. Licking a wrap at four in the morning. Terrified of sunrise but desperate to finish an idea. The idea itself is hazy. But exciting. Every cigarette pull like syrup for a clenched jaw. No thoughts just write write write. Smoke a spliff. Take the edge off. Wank myself to sleep. A merry-go-round of dicks and vaginas on my eyelids. Fake orgasms in my eardrums.

Thinking of women I could have booty called. But the writing was important. Next day I see someone. And I look fucked. LOOK WHAT I WROTE. LOOK WHAT I DID. LISTEN TO THIS. READ THIS. Undeniable. The joy that creating brings me. I didn't care how I'd got there or what it cost me. I'd made something and that was important. I think people around me could see that.

I was a functional cocaine abuser. I could go fucking anywhere. Family functions. Anywhere. If I was making music in the studio and that studio was in a family home and that session started at midday, I was doing lines in their toilet at eleven in the morning. Without getting high I felt muted. There were all these words I couldn't access. Or didn't know how to. I needed stimulants to speed through my doubt barriers. Without them it was all thought, no action.

But one morning before a midday studio session I snorted a couple of lines at my black dining table and then threw up. My whole body heated up. I instantly sweated profusely from every pore. And vomited. I looked at the remnants in the sink and thought, this isn't good. Should probably stop this.

After a trip to Brooklyn, I did. I didn't stop. I cut down. Significantly. Me and some friends escaped there. One friend of mine is a cool kid. He met other cool kids. It led to me staying with this girl. Cool kid. Small flat. She shared it with a person I've forgotten. They probably went to college together. Rats in the bins downstairs but cheap rent. Lent me a book about 'time'. She woke up one morning, popped open a plastic can of pills before she'd even washed her face. I asked what they were. She said

Adderall, it's for ADHD. Asked if I wanted some. I considered the fact I'd been diagnosed and hadn't paid it much attention. No harm. Considering the other shit I've been taking.

About forty minutes later my mind was blown. I had never been able to think about my thoughts before. To consider them. And here I was in a peaceful silence. Simply choosing not to say anything. Because I didn't want to. My friends kept asking if I was ok and I kept saying I was fine. With a childish grin and semi-low eyelids. My mind wasn't noisy. I wasn't impulsively saying and doing things. I asked my friends if it was usual to be able to think about what you say before you say it. Their response led me to believe I should give medication a go. And around that time, this hacker I know told me about Modafinil.

So I started self-medicating. With this Modafinil shit that I got off the internet. I don't think it was illegal but it should have been prescribed. And the effect it had on me was something else. I made beats. Wrote scripts. A fucking one-man show, almost. Treatments. Emails. I was a work machine. And I had no desire to do anything else. I just created and went wherever that took me. Started a collective. A group WhatsApp for that collective. Made the website in a day. Sorted everyone email addresses. Put on shows. It was fucking hectic. But it's all I cared about. I had no interest really in social situations or spending time on non-creative things. Everything was to be instant and transactional but with a sprinkle of spirituality. Bad boy Buddhist. Psychopath but Zen.

I'd freak out if the foil crinkled. If I couldn't feel a thick disc beneath my thumb and I'd forgotten to order any more. I'd panic. I didn't know who I was without that feeling. The rise into razor-sharp focus. I'd rummage through bags. Coat pockets. Check I hadn't left a loose one at the studio. Ravenous energy. I was sewn into that elevation. It threaded itself into my perception of the world. A needle prick, to puncture the monotony. Sitting down and attempting to create without it felt too risky.

A couple of years later I was rediagnosed with ADHD by a professional. I had to have a psych evaluation for a job I was doing. I was sat opposite this man, South Asian, alright suit, relaxing voice, in an office in central London. Where all the medical people are. Around Harley Street. So many objects in the office were made of a dark mahogany. Gave it a kind of esteem. Fortunately the chair wasn't. It was just a quite comfy office chair. Felt like I was blowing this guy's mind a bit.

He was very aware of how much I was swearing. Not that I was being offensive. Seemed impulsive to him. It is impulsive, but I love swearing. I was fidgety too. He did some other tests but the diagnosis was clear. He had ADHD too! Told me he was on the maximum amount of medication possible. Took it every morning, lasted twelve hours. Fascinating. He asked me if I had been self-medicating and I told him yes. Said I used to do loads of cocaine but I stopped and took Modafinil instead. He said Modafinil was an accepted form of medication and asked me how much I'd been taking. I said sometimes two tablets. He asked how strong one tablet was. I said 200 milligrams. Then he went silent. For quite a long time. Looked at me straight through his glasses. Went over it again. Verified it. He wanted to make sure he'd heard me right when I said I'd been taking 400 milligrams of Modafinil a day. I said yes. He said we need to get you an alternate prescription as soon as possible.

When I got the new medication, Concerta, I could see that each tablet was only 16 milligrams. I read the little leaflet that came with the bottle. It had a section called 'How To Know You've Overdosed'. To my amazement I read all the feelings I experienced on Modafinil when I thought it was kicking in. Sweating. High heart rate. Dry tongue. I'd been overdosing near enough every day for eighteen months.

Right now, I'm considering the chance that it could have played a part in this fuck-up. So I'm cutting it out. Cocaine and alcohol, I'm never fucking touching again. Weed I might need to.

*

Same walk as I did that night. Except it's daytime now. Don't feel like I'm being followed. Very alone. Green and yellow bushes. School kids. Skipping. I used to want to skip school. Craving it a little. In this moment. The safety of it. A few bus stops. People waiting. Big steps up to big houses. Roundabout with a little paradise in it. An island. Protected by oscillating vehicles. Can only journey to it at night. In the early hours. When there's no work. Middle of the afternoon now. I'm going to get my stuff. Got my letter in my hand. As well as her keys. She's got some stuff to give me. Going to swap and hope for the best.

Door opens. There she is. Cold. Beautiful. She's properly done her face up. Got a nice outfit on. Doesn't dwell.

Opens the door, walks back in, says her best mate is there. Makes sense, I suppose. They continue to talk and make food in the kitchen as if I'm not there. I walk into the bedroom and begin to grab my stuff.

Everything's familiar except the weight of the air. Something is repellent. It's undeniable. But I still want to hide under that duvet.

I walk into the kitchen and hand Chloe the letter along with her keys. I'm hoping she picks up on the fact that I've written one. She seems so grown up. Gigantic. Like she's grown a few inches. I maintain my composure. Can't be saying anything in front of her mate. Got to just leave. So I leave. Walk down the corridor. Don't look back. Out the door.

But I've made a mistake. I can't just go home. I have to add a link. Stay in touch somehow. Make a future out of this. Somehow. I press the buzzer. Dull thudding. Door opens. Unimpressed.

'Please can we just talk?'

'No.'

Pause. 'This is yours too.'

I hold my hands out. She drops something into them. The labradorite wolf necklace.

11

Punching Custard

Tai tells me again. Give it time. She'll come round. While putting food in the microwave. Special food made up only of nutrients. Perfect for training. Taste gets boring after a while but we just smother it in hot sauce. Ketchup. Whatever. Comfort food's the first sacrifice in terms of health. We live in a world of anti-life ingredients. The more I've learnt, the more paranoid I've become. I've got to stay clean and energised. I'm just happier that way. But I've got to fight the allure of fast food and quick fixes. Otherwise I can trip into that feedback loop. Fats and sugars. Instant joy. Grabbing the fat around my stomach isn't so sweet. Don't feel like eating at the moment anyway. Good thing Tai's here. He says I should train. He's right. And I will. We sit at the table. All I can think about is smoking. The clock behind him is broken. He reminds me he knows what it's like to be cheated on. She's angry. Let her be angry. But I can't believe she can just drop me like that, I say. Does she not love me any more? Did she ever love me? Of course she loves you! he says with a mouthful of food. I stare at the single grain of rice that's been propelled onto my hand from Tai's mouth. That's why she's angry, he says. It means she cares. Imagine what indifference would be like. Killer. I tell him I went and got my stuff. All the details. Gave me the necklace back. I understand what Tai's trying to say. Waiting seems unfeasible though. The pain needs to stop. It's as simple as that. Doesn't have to be like this. She'll read the letter at some point. I should start writing another one in more detail. More words. Real heart.

The next day I cycle to her house on my own, uninvited. I'm crying while cycling. I get there and turn straight around. Crying and cycling back. A group of builders watch me. Sad sight. Banter.

I work on this letter and pull in everything that kept us close. I focus in on tiny details. Minute moments of love and awareness. It's truly loving. To analyse, to pick up on things others drop. Specifically shine a light into the corners. It pays to pay attention. So I'm thinking of tiny things. Pretty marbles. Rounding up all my marbles. The way she says the word 'always'. Sounds like hallways. Why we work. Why I fucked up. Why I won't again. The great beyond. How incredible a second chance would be. Why I deserve a second chance. Why everyone deserves a second chance. I wonder if she's read the first letter. I text her. I ask if she's read it. She texts back. She doesn't want to speak to me. I get back to this new and much better letter. I should push weights at some point. My chest is tight.

Spooky action at a distance. Particles change when they're not observed. Maybe if I ignore the situation, she'd pay more attention. Undeniable. Impossible. This next letter is long. Detailed. I've put everything into it. We've been speaking via email. Feels less invasive. I decide the suggestion of space is mainly phone-based. Emails are easy to ignore. They're gentler. They have titles. Everyone uses full names. There's an air of romance too. A letter from war. Albeit self-inflicted.

Honestly, if she backs this off, I'll stop. But she's got to read it. I've put everything in it. Every day I'm self-editing. Removing anything risky. Re-reading, re-reading. Only danger with the written word is tone. I'm having to form sentences hoping they'll sound like a strong version of me. A mature, changed me. Even if it hasn't been that long. I can't have my tone of voice match the one she heard in the kitchen. Distant. Misguided. I'm betting she'll read the letter in that tone of voice.

And time continues to move like thick liquid. Like custard. If you dip a hand in custard, it's soft. If you punch it, it becomes rock solid. Right now it feels like I'm punching custard. I spend time trying to guess what she's thinking, what's she's doing. How to be one step ahead. What secret spice I can stick in a sentence. Add to the letter. Ultimate recipe. Send it off. Eventually I settle. Three pages long or something. I've read it back too many times. I click send and hear nothing. A little aeroplane noise and then fear. Can't unsend an email. Can't delete or edit. That's it. Can try and drown it in other emails. That's all. Coffee, thoughts, custard, patience, agony.

Days pass.

Days pass.

Days pass.

Chloe texts me. She's read the letter. The new one. The really long one. Says she'll meet me on Wednesday. A week from now.

My heart lights up. My body is full of energy. As if from nowhere, I've got a hold of some rope.

12

Who Am I to You?

I had been to see a therapist in Central London. Because of Chloe. She recommended one and I went for it. Felt like a long time coming. Needed it. Up until that point, whenever the image of me having a panic attack in an Airbnb in Milan, mid-argument with my ex Suzy, popped into my head I would think, I should probably have a look at that. There were many signs in that relationship that I needed therapy. I'm realising that more now. So once a week I've been turning a corner. Onto a street lined with black railings. Vegan café round the block. Every building looks professional. I never really see anyone but there's never a parking space. Not that I drive. Mostly jump out of Ubers in a fluster. Feathers everywhere. You hit the buzzer. She says come up. Up the stairs.

Sometimes you hear sobbing. Sometimes nothing. Toilets are the floor below the room. She's high up though. Feels like half the session is making it up there. The room is plain. Couple of paintings. Doubt they mean anything. Windows to the left. A sofa. Little table on the side with tissues and water. A little clock. My therapist likes to film the sessions, look back on them later. She charges her iPad, sits down in front of me. Giving away nothing. Calm. Stern. Perhaps a little underwhelmed by life. Burdened with understanding. She looks like a therapist. First session I bounced in. Toe tapping. Leg jiggling. Apologised for being late. She wouldn't respond.

'So . . . what are we going to talk about?'

And I talked. I'm good at talking. And she watched. Her eyes would dart around my body. She'd ask why I was so fidgety. ADHD, I would say, just who I am. She would ask if it was ADHD or anxiety. Would spin me out. Definitely ADHD, I would say. She'd ask why I was being defensive. I would say I wasn't. Then she would ask who she was to me.

'Who am I to you right now?' she would say. Like I'm supposed to know what the fuck that means.

'My therapist?' I would say.

'Am I?' she would say. Some kind of game, perhaps? Didn't feel very productive. Maybe I'd laugh it off. Try and move things on a bit. Felt like wasted time. Telling my therapist that I think she's my therapist. After a couple of sessions she concluded that I actually ran on anxiety. She told me that anxiety was my petrol. Followed up by asking if I really wanted to get into this. Warned that once we opened this box it would throw my life into the air. She didn't say that exactly. But I imagined it as such. Like my sense of self was lodged inside a confetti canon. And these sessions would consist of me picking up all the little multi-coloured pieces. Organising them by colour. Making sure I wasn't near a window on a windy day. I'd begun therapy before cheating on Chloe. But I didn't tell my therapist what I had done. I didn't ask her if I should say anything.

My sessions are often in the dark now that it's winter. And they've taken a turn since my life has imploded. Chloe has done therapy. So at the last couple of sessions I've fantasised that she might even be in the same building. Telling her therapist what a piece of shit I am. Or, worse, having her therapist confirm it. On the way up the stairs I wonder how I'd feel if I bumped into her. Lock eyes in the doorway. I walk slowly out of these sessions and convince myself life will push us back together. But it never happens. I considered standing outside all day in case she showed up. Even in this state, I knew that was too far. I must admit I wasn't able to think of much else.

I thought I was a feminist. I thought I respected the concept of space. Understood that you had to let women come to their own conclusions. But I'd never anticipated being in this space. And I'm sure Chloe is wrong about me. I'm sure she's not thinking straight.

And now that I'm seeing her next week, life tastes different. The air is edible. Hope-flavoured sandwiches. I'm primed. I've got the plate spinning. Now I just want to do a few tricks to prove my balance. This pain of the last couple of weeks means everything. I'm completely different now. I'm a new leaf. Veins throbbing with promise. I'm the exception to the rule. People say that people don't change. That you can't come back from this. I have to prove that you can. First thing I have to do is appear completely fine. As if this whole situation hasn't obliterated me.

Then I'm going to spend hours making a meticulous t-shirt design of a cat. I'm going to draw the cat, scan it into the computer, make it into a graphic and then get it printed high quality. No shitty stuff. The best quality.

Oversized. So she can wear it to bed. She'll know that love and time has gone into it. That says something. Tai agrees, and he's a proper romantic. Thoughtful behaviour always wins. I'm also going to get a butterfly tattoo. Because I feel as though right now I'm breaking out of my cocoon. It's this exact fuck-up that's given me the strength to break free of myself. Tai doesn't argue it.

A few days later I'm sat over a chair in my flat. In reverse. Like a Britney Spears video. I know this tattoo artist called Thea. From Plymouth. Friends with my other friend who's got loads of tattoos. She's down for visits. And she's here now. In the past everyone's ended up getting tattoos. I've got Jake's handwriting all over me. Mine on him too. Just me today though. The sun's shining. I'm topless. Good music playing. Chain smoking as usual. Zoning out to the hum. The Hummingbird is singing. It's singing and signing my arm. The pain makes my mouth water but I like it. Especially right now. Feels like I deserve it. And I've needed a rush of endorphins. I ask Tai to take a picture and post it. I put sunglasses on. Poker face and it's done. I look cool as fuck. He posts it. Does she see it? She must be thinking about how cool and romantic that is. Surely.

I walk into my local pub. The Chamber. Upper middle-class. Fancy beers. I've had a few birthdays here. Feels homely. I know the owner. Great chef. Does this thing called 'Chef's Table' where everyone wears headphones and he creates a dessert in time to music. That was one of my favourite birthdays. After I ate the dessert I got really hyperactive and passed out twenty-five minutes later. Used to come in here to meet my dealer too before he was banned. The woman I see working here the most is Danish. Walks with a slight limp. I don't know how old she is but she isn't young. Which is kind of wonderful because she seems young. If that makes sense.

My neighbour Lucy is here. The one I see smoking spliffs and miming to her boyfriend. Who she recently broke up with. Spoken to her a bit about it. Was much more confident in my advice prior to this situation. I've texted her a few times and she's been helpful. She kind of knows Chloe. That's the only problem. And the temptation to have her intervene is too high. She thinks things will turn around. But also that cheating sucks. Everyone seems to agree about that. She wonders if she would have even wanted to know. Another point of contention.

Lucy is standing at the bar with another blonde woman. This one a little shorter. Bright blue eyes. Striking face. Scandinavian. Don't even have to ask. Never met her before. Lucy introduces us. Her name's Amalie. They're on their way out, but I tell Lucy that things are looking up. Going to speak to Chloe next Wednesday. Good luck, she says. Big smile. I think Amalie waved.

Conquering women is a common theme in romantic comedies. No one questions it. Silver-screen leeway. And men usually write the scripts. So eventually the women 'give in'. Or are overcome with how 'flattering' persistence is. But I've heard different from the women around me. Some of them anyway. Sometimes they actually just don't want to see or speak to you. And anything past that is abusive. I'd agree. And then we'd think about films like *Love Actually*. When that guy stalks his best mate's wife for an entire film and then traps her at her door and kisses her and then tells himself he's going to stop stalking her. Or the hundred films when a guy plays a guitar at a window. Or writes someone's name in the clouds with a fucking plane. It's always about making someone change their mind. Felt ridiculous. But I'm in the middle of it. Drowning in potential big gestures. Trying not to text Chloe every single fucking day. Or email her. Or some form of contact. Never thought I'd empathise with male protagonists in romantic comedies though. People say the heart wants what it wants. I can't think of anything other than getting Chloe back. That's what it really, really wants. Spice Girl energy.

I'm on Photoshop designing the t-shirt I'm going to give to Chloe when I see her. The design will blow her away. I'm creating a collage using photos that we'd taken together and images that she loves. Collages are romantic. A mosaic of musings. Surely everyone wants to be a muse? I'm not sure actually. I wrote about Suzy a lot. Even when we weren't together. Especially when we weren't together. Some of the best writing I've ever done. Always positive. Always about loving her. Not being good enough for her. But I wasn't loving enough in the actual relationship. And I think she would have preferred that. My friends at the time would tell me that she was the one. That I was bound to her. Muse or not, the spark went elsewhere. I wrote a couple of things about Chloe but the desire had passed. As the months went on my mind got fuzzy. But now – now she's all I can think about. And she's the muse. I've always been into graphic design. I used to make MySpaces for money as a teenager. Kept me going. I knew how to write code. Thankfully I still know enough to do this collage. I want my effort as a neon sign. Unmissable. No bullshit. I'm better than all the men before. Other men don't design collages and print a single high-quality t-shirt. They don't write three-page letters binding romance to numerology. This is proof that I'm stepping up. Tai agrees. He knows this about me. I adapt quickly. I rise to the occasion. And this won't be any different.

I've learnt my lesson. I know what Chloe deserves. This shit's going down in history. We're going to make up and be together forever. This woman will have appreciated my honesty. Her forgiveness will create an infinite chain. A love formed in a shadow. The highest form of embrace. Tai says he'll come with me to the t-shirt design place when I'm done. Down Ladbroke Grove.*

---

* Yes, I'm living in a dream world.

13

The Corners of the Painting

Portobello Road. The market. Shouting and screaming. Fish and fruit. All types of clothing. Every shade of skin. All hustle. Barking and biting. Schmoozy and poor. Starts off rough, ends up swanky. One road. Been coming here since childhood. Loved the array. The multiple choices. Variation. Trinkets and treasures. Bought a jade necklace here once. Treasured it. Had a dragon on it. Used to love dragons as a kid. Fell in love somewhere between mythology and SisQó. I got my nose pierced here with Jake. By a woman nicknamed the Queen of Portobello. She said, 'On the count of three,' and then pierced my nose instantly. If there's ever a time to lie to a person, it's then. Tai and I find a little place to have lunch before I go and get the t-shirt printed. Artisan bakery. Unhealthy but looks healthy. Looks divine. And well-mannered. This place looks like a polite person.

'You don't fancy a croissant?'

'It's one of the worst things you can eat.'

'But they're so tasty.'

'All of the worst stuff is tasty.'

'I think I want to be super fit just so I can eat croissants.'

'You can eat a croissant now! You're in good shape! Just don't eat like six a day.'

I grab the fat around my stomach. I could eat six a day. I walk up to the till. Buy us both coffees. Buy myself a croissant. Sit back down. Eat the croissant. Offer some to Tai.

'Nah, I'm good, bro. I'm already dealing with a dad bod at the moment.'

Tai is muscly and more defined than anybody I know. Maybe anybody in the world.

'You're kidding?'

'Nah, man, it's all relative. My fat might be your thin. And vice versa.'

'What?'

I finish the last bit of my croissant. I stick a few flakes to my finger. Shove them in too. Inspect my lips with tongue. 'Do you think this is going to work?'

'I think she'll forgive you, yeah.'

'Really?'

'Yeah. She just needed a bit of time to understand. You're a special guy, you know. And it's clear that you know you were stupid.' Tai pauses. But not for long. 'Why do you think you did it?'

'Did what?'

'Cheat on her. Why did you do it?'

I breathe out. 'I never meant to cheat on her, man. I just wanted to destroy myself.'

'Just total self-sabotage?'

'Yeah, pretty much. But never again. I never want to feel like this again.'

*

Sadness and time are lethal. But I'm keying into the little version of me as much as possible. I close my eyes and see that he's eating apple pie. I text Jessica and tell her. She's into it. Heading down Westbourne Grove to get my bike fixed. Look at some art. Bowling with Jake and Tai later. And Jake's girlfriend, Tanya. She's been a saving grace. Very good at organising. Recovering drug addict. Likes to keep herself on the move.

I walk into a gallery on the Grove. And stare at these shapes. Art's supposed to make you feel. Something I learnt not long ago. Didn't understand it for a long time. Loved Monet as a kid. The colours mainly. Turquoise shades. Oversized lily pads. Lost touch as I grew older. Like many people I know. Thought it was for fancy people. At least, understanding it was. I did enjoy art in school. Took it as a GCSE. But ended up throwing my work at the teacher and getting an E. Not a fan of authority. My breakthrough with art was picturesque. I was on holiday in Miami with some friends. An art festival supposedly, but art wasn't on the pallette. That's not why we were there. Instead it was another blank canvas to be splattered with drugs. Cocaine and alcohol as usual. Vibrant. I arrived jetlagged. Drunk a whole bottle of Jägermeister, did a somersault on the bed and passed out. Was woken up some time later with three white slugs. Powdered nose and I was ready to party. Got to the party and someone gave me what I thought was ecstasy. Turns out it was a Valium and I passed out again. On the second night out I was introduced to a woman.

Friend of a friend. Blonde, red lipstick, blue eyes. Messy. The introduction was electric. Touched hands and felt something. Bizarre. Just knew we were going to be close. And we were. For the remaining time. Sat on the beach and watched people dance around a fire. Rich people. People with time and money. She was a painter herself. Studied in London. Had a few mutuals but she was American. All American. Loose white shirt. We kissed but nothing more. I wanted more for sure. I lost her at one point and ended up walking back to my hotel room alone. Locked out. Sank down next to the door. Day after that, her and I went to visit the main gallery. I was still getting my head around the fact it was an art festival. They checked our bags as we walked in. The day before, two people working at the gallery had got into a fight and one person started stabbing the other with a scalpel. Took ages till somebody intervened because people thought it was a performance piece.

We walked up to a huge mural. An artist had drawn two skeletons getting out of a car. The detail was awesome. Eight or nine people were photographing it. I said, 'Woah.' And she said, 'Ugh, I hate it.' I was lost. 'How can you hate that?' I said. 'It's so detailed.' She didn't respond. I said, 'You don't have to like it but you've got to appreciate the skill?' She shifted weight onto her hip, looked me dead in the eyes and asked why. 'Art isn't about being good at drawing,' she said. 'It's about how it makes you feel.'

From that point life was different. Maybe I understood why people swam around exhibitions with their hands behind their backs. They were pushing out their organs. Lessening the obstruction between their bodies and the work. Still unacceptable to wear a thin scarf in summer but the rest made sense. I stood in front of pieces from then. And decided in moments whether or not I enjoyed them. One exhibition I walked into and walked straight out. 'Ugh, I hate it,' I thought.

She ended up teaching me how to paint. In an abandoned warehouse in downtown LA. Very cinematic. Cigarettes and acrylics. Wine and oil. She told me to never look at what I was drawing. Only the object. To trust that my hand would know what to do. She would appear over my shoulder and breathe encouragement. Exactly what I needed. I painted my first picture that trip. It was of a photo I took on my phone. Random guy sat in a car shielding himself from the sun with a book. While also wearing sunglasses. I found that interesting. Painted it. Felt a sense of achievement. She was telling me I could be a painter. Great eye for colour. The encouragement made my soul sing. Built my confidence. Like I was back on the council estate handing my mum a drawing. I'd discovered a new passion. And I'm forever thankful. Nothing more ever came of that relationship. Partly 'cause we lived thousands of miles from each other. Mostly because of the chasm of cultural differences. And she was fucking intense. Maybe I led her on. Maybe I'm intense.

Right now in this West London gallery, devoid of encouragement, this art's not doing much for me. I just find myself drawn to the corners. Wondering if anyone cares about them. One of these pieces is cool. Has Chloe's favourite colours on it. It's four hundred pounds. I buy it. Can add that to the love package. Strengthen the recovery.

14

A Week After

Whoever designed bowling shoes is a clown. I don't wear them. This alley doesn't give a fuck. Thank God. They do help with slide or whatever but no thanks. And they stink. No one can bowl properly anyway. My technique is all over the place. Might be something to do with being left-handed. I put my first two fingers in, chuck the ball and end up in a Spider-Man stance. Jake's decided to throw the game by attempting to emulate pros and spin the ball. To be fair, when he gets some curve on it, it's impressive. Tai is the best. Probably all the muscles. Gets five strikes or something. Jake's girlfriend Tanya is shit. She doesn't care though. So in a way she always wins. Nothing beats a good loser. I can be way too competitive. Christmases have been ruined. If I lose, it's hell. A tsunami of disappointment. My parents always watched me play football in my early teens. I'd cry after matches sometimes. Not because we lost. Just because I didn't score. My team could win and I would still cry.

That competitive energy is a massive part of who I am today. Blessing and a curse. I am not Tanya. I am not a good loser. There's an alternate reality where I've taken everything in my stride. Unbothered. Unflappable. Chin up, keep it moving. Just another loss. I do not live in that reality. Right now I am not there. I'm fighting.

I think about what I'm going to say to Chloe when I see her. She's going to be angry. But the t-shirt and the artwork mixed with my regret will shift things. Would she have agreed to meet if a part of her didn't believe in me?

My favourite film is *Space Jam*. Absolute classic. Not a single cartoon or animated character has outdone Bugs Bunny's performance in that film. The moral of the film is to believe in the impossible. To look beyond the confines of '3D Land'. Michael Jordan, the star of the film, realises this at the very end. When he's got these three monsters stopping him from scoring a basket during an intergalactic basketball game. He extends his arm. Stretches his imagination. Frees himself from convention. I like the idea that love is like that stretch. To be a partner whose arms can travel through physics. Cradle someone at their lowest in belief of their future.*

We all go our separate ways after bowling. Tanya and Jake hop in an Uber. I order one and light a cigarette. Lean against a glass window. Ice on the back of my head. Short breathing. It's drizzling. Not heavy enough to be rain but enough to put your hood up.

I whip my phone out. Go through the motions. We've all got our go-to phone taps. Whatever apps provide promise. Quick refresh potential present. Infinite Christmas. Social media's usually high up there. Keeping up with what's going on. Email's last for me. Self-employed. Signed up to way too many newsletters. Hotel offers. Cafés selling

---

* Yes, 'potential' is problematic.

my data and shit. I get to it. My email says 'loading messages'. This time it's no business. Chloe's name is at the top.

I open up the email. The title is 'Letter'. My heart drops. Why's she emailing me a letter now? Just before we're supposed to meet? In the email is a photograph of a letter Chloe has written. She's changed her mind about seeing me. Short. Concise. Handwritten. It reads as an acknowledgement of my efforts but a disbelief in my intentions. Good luck but fuck off, basically. My ears start ringing.

*

I'm on the phone to my friend Gabriella. I fell in love with her when I was 18 but it didn't work out. Became friends instead. She's straight-talking. Driven. Puts me in my place. I'm outside my flat. Heart jumping like rainwater on the tarmac. In a spin. Wrong way round a roundabout. This has not gone my way. This isn't supposed to happen. Chloe was not supposed to change her mind. I had everything ready. I had the words. The painting. The t-shirt. What the fuck? The outside light I'm stood underneath feels harsh. Gabriella isn't having it either. No bubble wrap, no sugar-coating. She holds the opposing reality. I've lost. I've lost it. I'm protesting again.

'I don't even understand why this is such a big thing! I didn't even fuck anyone else. I just got a blowjob. What about everything else that's good about me? Is that not enough? If this was the other way around, I would NEVER do this. I don't even understand why we have a society that encourages this kind of behaviour. We're encouraged to be so possessive over another person's body. It's honestly so—'

'You need to listen—'

'—so ridiculous. Like, if you think about it, the person isn't even there when cheating happens. Do you know what I mean? How can something that a person is in no way physically there for have such a detrimental effect? I get sexual health or whatever. I do get that. But what else is it? People are willing to just let love crumble because they can't deal with their own imagination? Come on, man. What the fuck!'

'SHUT THE FUCK UP AND LISTEN. You have no idea what it feels like to be cheated on—'

'That's not true—'

'I'm talking about adult years. We're adults now, ok! And you can't gallivant around talking about how people should and shouldn't feel about cheating! How dare you?! A lot of emotional stuff doesn't make any fucking sense but it still happens. A lot of people probably wish they didn't feel how they felt but they still do. Chloe has made her decision whether you like it or not, and to be honest it's not that outrageous because you have BETRAYED HER.'

'But you know me, man, I fucked up. That's not who I am.'

'Listen, we're not talking about me or what I know about you. I'm just making you aware that there's nothing you can do at this point. Leave her the fuck alone.'

I am fucking fuming. Brain buzzing. Panic insurgence. Got to get control of the wheel. Steer back onto the road.

I think about going over to Chloe's. Telling her to her face that she's wrong. She's only doing this because we haven't had a chance to speak. But something stops me. Feels like a step too far. Most painful no I've ever had.

15

When It Happened

They say that a tie perfectly encapsulates a man. One end a noose around the neck. The other end pointing to the penis. I cheated on my girlfriend Chloe at a wedding. Loads of ties, loads of dresses. Formless friendships. Familiar shapes and prickly pastimes. I've known the bride and groom since I was a teenager. Stomping round Brighton with baggy trousers and cans of cider. Back when I could get pissed for two pound fifty. Back when 'love' was disgusting.

The wedding was in a field. Big canopy. No service. Moon was half lit. Bright. I felt lost. In a sea of everyone. Two weeks prior to this I had taken cocaine for the first time in months. Thought I had a lid on it. I'd got myself to a place of moderation. Sensible choices. Chloe had been invited to a weekend away, in the countryside, with all her posh mates. The plan lodged in my chest immediately. But I couldn't break it down. Get the truth out of my mouth. Articulate my fears. It was a struggle. Didn't want to let her down. So instead I went along with it. Let it settle. Let the excitement build. Until the Wednesday before. I coughed. Not literally. We were laying on her bed watching something. As we often did. Telly at the end of the bed which I wasn't used to. Never had a telly in my room. Figured it would stop me sleeping. But a lot of people do. The words spluttered out of my mouth like I'd been resuscitated on a beach.

'I don't wanna go,' I said. No warning. Just that.

'What? What do you mean?'

'This weekend. I don't think I should go. I don't think it's a good idea.'

'What?! No! Why are you saying this now?'

I'm still horizontal. Freaking out. Then would have been a perfect time to explain why I didn't think it was a good idea, but I didn't. Too afraid of being a disappointment. I should have said I was worried about taking drugs. That a bunch of posh kids having a party in the countryside meant there would 100 per cent be cocaine. And if I'm there, surrounded by people I don't know, with no way of escaping, I would almost certainly end up doing that coke. And that wouldn't be a good idea. Because I was feeling unstable as it was. The honeymoon phase had ended and I was drowning in baggage. And cocaine was an old lover. That I had tussled with too many times. Kicked the habit more than once. Chloe didn't do drugs so it wouldn't be a joint thing. Not that that made it any better. Being around people high on cocaine while not high on cocaine is one of my top ten worst social experiences.

I explained nothing. Remained frozen. Took a moment. Changed my mind. Agreed to go with her to her friend's party. And then there I was. Surrounded by wealth and affluent offspring. Sore brown thumb. Sat at dinner. Most of my attention was on fitting in. Making jokes. Asking questions. My usual tactics. I was taught to work rooms from an early age. I can appear confident when terrified. At ease when unnerved. Part of the reason I'm successful Still spinning.

The dinner ended and people syphoned off into different rooms. There were so many different rooms. Outhouses. Guest houses. Attics. It was a barn conversion. Dreamlike. Fireplaces and shit. They didn't even live here, the family. The parents were there. Chloe's friend's parents. Spoke to them for five seconds. Wine was opened. A few jokes and they fucked off. Then the drugs came out.

I got friendly with this one guy who was a DJ. I think they all wanted to be DJs but he actually was one. Fluffy blonde hair. Glasses. Tall and a bit chubby. Lovable. Worked at an internet radio station. We had a bit in common. He had good taste in music. Common accent. I attached myself to him. We had a cigarette outside at the same time. Eventually he asked me if I wanted to go upstairs and do some coke. I took a look around the people I was with. All the different groups. Clusters of confusion. Spheres I didn't understand. Links I had spent a life away from. Chloe was somewhere with the people she was better friends with. So I accepted the invite. Hoping the rush would make things easier. Forgetting in a second all the complications that come with being high. Where my mind goes. My poor jaw muscles.

Once I came back from doing the line, Chloe wanted to have a word with me. I wasn't spending enough time with her. She wondered why I was being distant. Couldn't see the child in my eyes. Circling the playground. Looking for friends. Or perhaps, I couldn't see the child in hers.

Wondering why her partner had slipped away. Wandered into the woods and reappeared with glazed eyes and twigs in his hair.

There was a bit more fun the next day. Played rounders. Carried on drinking. I got beaten at table tennis. Felt off-centre but went along with it. Light bonds. Chloe seemed happier in the light of day. I had tied an internal balloon tight enough to last through the evening. But the next morning I woke up and it popped. Broke down entirely.

I sat on Chloe's bed, belly sobbing. Kept on saying, 'I don't know how to look after myself.' She was about to leave for work. I hadn't timed it very well. Made her late. Honestly, I'm glad she waited up. I was in pieces. Didn't understand why I had put myself through that. Why I couldn't stand up for myself. Make better decisions.

From then on the box was open. Pandora's one or whatever. Seashells on the top and shit. Tumbling through a void with drugs as a rope swing. I had no idea how to deal with any of it. All I knew at that point was destruction. Self-destruction. Annihilation.

And Chloe was away with friends this time without me. So at the haunted wedding reception with no phone reception, full of ghosts, my tummy tightened. I took pictures on my point-and-shoot camera to keep myself busy. Nikon 35ti. Bought in New York. Great flash apparently. But a lens didn't provide much of a barrier. Not really. The time between photos grew as the night when on. Every click, another step along the plank. I felt so far away from everyone. Our friend Scarlett sang as the bride and groom had their first dance. And all I could think about was how long it'd been since she and I had spoken on the phone. We used to be good friends.

I tried not to drink too much at the wedding. Initially. Or do drugs. Knowing my mindstate. Friends would wiggle their hands in front of their face at me and I'd shake my head. But this conversation with Mitchell. Started out ok. We'd spoken a little bit about my recent shock. My struggle to remain standing once the honeymoon period crashed. He picked up on it. I'd say something deep, then make a joke, keep it moving. I wanted to talk about him being a dad, hype him up about it, and I did. Lamented on how transcendent the experience will be. He's less expressive than me. Internalises most of his strong feelings. Half grinned between tokes of his cigarette. But there was another question weighing on my mind. Because I knew the answer. But I had to ask.

'Who's the godfather?' I asked.

'John, obviously,' he said.

Obviously. It was obvious. I knew that. They were best friends. But it hurt. Because we used to be best friends. And I wondered if all that we'd been through would engulf our recent silence. But that was hopeful. It made sense that it was John.

'Course,' I said.

And we carried on talking. But a part of me had muted. Everything else was a murmur. The conversation was a television in the other room. I got another hand signal over Mitchell's shoulder. This time I nodded. Yes please I'd like a drink. And some MDMA.

*

An hour later I couldn't feel the MDMA. So I took more. And then resorted to coke. As usual. And then word came that we were all hopping in cabs to end the night partying at a hotel. A hotel with cute little bathrooms.

Quirky hotel by the sea. Themed rooms. Psychedelic decor. Friend behind the bar so it was going off. Everything was a lot closer. The groups that were sporadically spread around the field were nearer each other. I knew I'd fucked it. I was in no position to make good decisions. So I had to be invisible. I tiptoed between sitting on a stall, smoking outside and snorting upstairs. A plan had been made with my friend Molly for us all to get a cab back to London at half one in the morning. That was the plan. All I had to do was not get into any trouble until then. Having a goal made the mental warfare easier. My mind had simplified, as it does when high, into three desires. More drugs, more booze and sex. Usually I have hundreds of thoughts. Having only these few is a twisted freedom.

I imagine my unconscious as a towering building. Something you'd see in Canary Wharf. I only ever experience a single floor. Full of glass rooms. Glass rooms teeming with familiar faces. Alternate versions of myself. The largest room occupied by my ego. The head honcho. Tailored suit. Sunglasses. Full of shit. Always nearest to the phone that leads up to head office. Guarding it. In the smallest room is my authentic self. The voice that needs to be heard. He wakes up surrounded by papers. Wondering how long he's been asleep. Ears piercing with the sound of a fire alarm. Chaos ensues. Through the office window he watches as people sprint down the hallway screaming. An alternate me wearing matching tropical shorts and shirt is on fire. Belting for the exit. My authentic self pops his head out of the office door and catches the eye of the ego. Stood completely still at the furthest end of the corridor. Sunglasses on. Totally black. Big grin. Massive cigar.

I decided that I fancied a woman in a red dress. You couldn't make it up. It was red, fitting, alluring. A fancy candle. She was sat with people I kind of knew, but I caught her eyes briefly and I couldn't stop thinking about it. I'd never met her before. My only goal was to not look at her again before half one. Every five minutes I checked the time on my phone. When I went out for a cigarette I saw a woman called Rachel talking to her ex-boyfriend James. I know her full name because I fantasised about her in school, endlessly. Beautiful. Elusive. It was the elusiveness that really did it. She didn't jump on social media in the same way as everyone else. So seeing her in person was extra special. She probably just hated social media. But it was genius. All her boyfriends looked the same. Lanky white boys. Nothing like me. Not a lead singer type but definitely friends with the band. I found it difficult knowing that not one part of my natural look fitted the bill. An unrequited obsession. I said hi and smoked. Got back inside. Checked the time.

At one fifteen in the morning, Molly told me that the plan was cancelled. Everyone had decided to stay out that night. Get the train back together in the morning. To Molly this was minor. She told me and bounced away. I was already slouching on my stool. Didn't move. Struggled to compute the situation. Figured I had to find somewhere to stay. But if there was any chance of being sensible, the unimaginable happened. Scarlett, our friend who had sung earlier at the wedding, tapped me on the shoulder and asked me if I'd met her friend, June. I straightened up and looked right into the eyes of the woman in the red dress. Smiling. Red lipstick to match the dress. Hi, I said. Ok great, Scarlett said and bounced off like Molly. Didn't want to be rude. We spoke for a bit longer. Then she sat down. Then we spoke more. Had more in common. But I knew I was in danger. So I was standoffish. Short, polite responses. Which had the opposite effect. She asked more questions. Seemed intrigued. The topic of a place to stay that night came up. Said she had an Airbnb round the corner. Was just her. Said she had a sofa. I thought, sure. I could sleep on the sofa. Wake up the next day and meet everyone. Great idea. No risks.

At her place. After having had a cigarette and a herbal tea. While making a bed of the sofa. She asked me an important question. She asked me if I had come with a 'plus one'. I knew what she meant. A part of me did. But it was too vague. There was too much space. I said I hadn't come with anyone. Which was a truthful response to the question. But a lie. It's not what she was asking. But it didn't fucking matter because I knew. And I lied. And worse. She slipped back into the living room half an hour later and said I could sleep in the bed. Said it was more comfortable. And I did. Because I was high. And I'm an idiot.

We lay on separate sides. Then got closer. Then a little closer. Too close, magnetically. I short-circuited. Became overwhelmed with possibility. Golden rule for addicts. Keep temptation away. I don't think I'm a sex addict. I'm a self-destruction addict. Don't eat the apple. Don't eat the cake. I've got a cousin with OCD who has to brush fire alarms with his finger. Turns out I like prodding them. As if there's a prize. Thankfully I didn't get that far. We ended up spooning. She spun round. Kissed me dramatically. We touched each other. She used her mouth. I lost my head. Didn't go any further though. She asked me if I had a condom and I didn't. A dead lifeline. This wasn't premeditated. My chest tightened like a tornado. The whirlwind subsided and I nestled into the debris. Heart leaking. Guilt, shame, confusion. One moment and everything's fucked.

The next morning I stared at the ceiling knowing my universe had collapsed. I needed a time machine. I was sober and aware. An irreversible taste. I say I was sober. Drugs have half-lives. I was uncomfortable. Twisted. June was still asleep. I had to escape. One of those sneak-outs. Like in the films. Redressed myself quietly. Felt odd getting back into a suit. At this time. First thing in the morning, like I was heading to the office. Very little going on in my head office other than more flames. More bedlam. But funnelled into a singular, tortuous feeling. A monotonous hum. There's a Japanese idiom 'mono no aware'. It translates literally as 'the pathos of things' or 'an empathy towards things'. It speaks of the awareness of impermanence. A deep, gentle sadness that comes with acknowledging that transience is the permanent state of being.

But I can't say I felt that way. Nothing gentle about it. Everything's been torn apart.

*

Next day I sat on a bus with sick in my mouth. Chloe was still away on holiday. What's worse is that she was away celebrating a job she just got. Girls' holiday but to mark an event. And while they clinked glasses and ate dessert I was eating chemicals and breaking trust. I was staring out the front of the top deck. Whirring trees. Twigs slapping the plastic windows. I was thinking about damage control. Trying to be objective. Wondering if my error could end there. Memory erased. Guilt swallowed.

My mate phoned me. 'Heard you were a naughty boy last night,' he said.

'Yeah,' I said.

That was all. His tone was jokey, mine wasn't. In fairness fucking up wasn't alien to us. That particular friend, Piers. He fucked up all the time. So much so that we tried to stage an intervention once. Suggested he stop cheating on his girlfriend. He was the worst version of himself back then. He'd cheat yet act insanely jealous. Toxic as fuck. But it all stemmed from somewhere. I know where. His parents. And a parent he didn't get to choose. Difficult to know where the buck stops. Hurt people hurt people. We're all carrying shit. Out of all of my friends I think Piers and I shared that coupling with chaos the most. Battling with our shadows. We'd even go for the same women. We look completely different, but our pain's a similar colour. Sometimes I'd tell a joke and no one in the room would find it funny but him.

I remember looking out of the bus window and seeing Molly. Smile blossomed. Her disposition beat her hangover. Waved excitedly at me. I waved back. Wondered if she knew.

16

Three Weeks After

'Chloe keeps liking all of my photos on Instagram. It's weird.'

Me and my neighbour Lucy are at her dining table. Smoking. Drinking herbal teas. She's studying art and has a great eye for decor. Muted pastels mainly. Art hung sparingly. Every piece is good. She models too. Got a great face. Eyes especially. Huge smile. Purely platonic with us. I can't stand how she eats.

'Would you be doing this? If this had happened to you? Would you react like this?'

'Umm . . . well, I think I'd take into account that it was only a blowjob for sure.'

Exactly what I want to hear.

'Why can't I get her to listen to me then? Just hear me out?'

'Yeah . . . I don't know. I think you just have to let her do her thing for a bit.'

Not what I want to hear. I don't want her to do her thing for a bit. I want to be forgiven immediately. This is fucked. No one seems to understand the gravity of the situation. And it can't be fixed instantly, which is wild.

There isn't a heartbreak pill or a course of anti-youfuckedits that will subside misery in seven days. I've got to sit in this. 'And what am I supposed to do?'

'I don't really know. Sorry. Feel it all, I suppose. It'll get better.'

'Should I be trying to move on? Fuck someone else?'

'Well . . . I probably wouldn't do that any time soon, no. Not if you want her back.'

'And she's speaking to you?'

'Seems to be.'

'Why don't you tell her you think this is all bullshit? Have my back or whatever?'

'You really want me to do that?'

'Yeah?'

'I mean . . . I will if you really want me to. I actually was wondering if I could ask her a question about work though. She's got a contact I need . . .'

Doesn't feel like Lucy's getting it. Or maybe she is and feels uncomfortable. No one can see that I'm bleeding everywhere. Or hear the endless conference behind my eyes. Maybe I don't look that different. Calm, together. I haven't cried in front of Lucy. Maybe that would change things. Chloe messaging her hurts. I can feel her energy everywhere. We live so close to each other. Every day is a possible opportunity to bump into each other. Which means that every day that doesn't happen feels punishing. I need to be away from memories and currents and faded fingerprints. Finding friends on the other side of London won't do it.

*

I'm leaving the country. I've got a contact at an airline who got me a concession ticket. I paid a couple of grand for it. Means I can book a flight at any moment and fly business. Everyone who works as a host or hostess gets one apparently. One concession ticket so they can book their friends, partners or family on flights. But some of them think *fuck that* and sell it. They're not allowed to. But I've got one. Right now it's perfect. I've got an uncle in Brazil. I'll just fly away and stay with him if he's ok with it. Haven't seen him since I was 15. Brazil is really far. Six thousand miles or something. Pain's got to hurt less that far away. In the heat.

Heathrow. Middle of the day. It's sunny, bright and vast. A lot of baggage. Overwhelmed by opportunity. Everyone's disappearing. Running. Returning. You can go anywhere. I feel like a tiny dot. I want to be bigger. Or know more. Some people are pushing trolleys with purpose. They know where the tin bird flies. They've seen it all. Or they're just getting on with it. So many legs going in different directions. Lives that span the globe. I wonder how many of these people are lost, or heartbroken. Or have been. And know exactly where I should go. Everyone's the centre of their own universe, aren't they?

I'm nervous checking in, in case this ticket situation fucks up. Woman at the desk is sweet. Smiles at me and says they can't allocate a seat until check-in closes. Says she'll bump me up to business if possible. Twenty minutes later the ticket's printed. Business it is. That's a win. Now I feel special. Best bit of business class is the lounge. Free food. Free coffee. I can't get that council-estate mentality out of my head. If it's free, I'll take it. Can't turn it down if it's free. When I've attended parties before with free drinks, it's got out of hand. At a party in Primrose Hill, someone stupid rich, his patio turned into a swimming pool. Fuck knows how I ended up there. One of the toilets was hidden in a bookcase. You had to push the bookcase and there was a secret door. I lost my vision at that party after an hour.

They're not letting me into the business lounge. I keep showing them that I'm sitting in business, but they're saying I don't have the right ticket. The woman looks concerned. Mixed-race, glasses, curly hair pulled back, big cheeks. What's the female equivalent of avuncular? She's that. I figure I've got to leave it and ring my connect. I walk away and dial the number.

'Yo, you alright?'

'Dude, they're not letting me into the business lounge.'

'What! Nooo! Mate, you can't go to the business lounge. Fuck.'

'Oh, really?'

'Nah, that's not part of it. Fuck. Are you there now?'

'Well, I've walked off now.'

'Ok, don't go back. That's not how this works. You've got to keep your head down. Concession tickets aren't allowed in the lounge, and we have to keep this under the radar. If they start reporting that concession passes are turning up asking for entry, bro, this whole thing gonna get blown wide open.'

'Alright, alright. My bad. I didn't know. It should be ok. I'll go sit somewhere else.'

'This concession ticket shit is seriously against policy. The whole thing'll get fucked up.'

'I got it.'

Gutted about that. Having to buy my own croissants. I wander around duty free. I see her scent. Heart trips. Fumbles. All the adverts remind me of her. All the women posing. Seducing. They're all her. And I'm me. In a camouflage tracksuit. Can't get into the business lounge. I want to be an advert. Looking my best. Muscles bulging. I'm in good shape but I don't feel it. I'm actually in amazing shape but it doesn't matter. More out of anxiety than anything. More out of a desperation to be as attractive as possible. Just in case that makes any kind of difference. I haven't got any panic spare for my body right now. I pinch my stomach and flex my chest without thinking. But it's all unconscious. I've learnt you have to keep moving, keep pushing. Otherwise it all gets clogged up. And the anxiety is constant. Surging through me. Plugged into an infinite supply. I just want to turn it off. At the mains. But that's not how it works. And if my mind's anything to go by. I better stay in shape. Because I'm constantly thinking about how attractive I find Chloe.

I sit at a café and start mapping out another letter. Text a friend. Pray that Chloe finds out I'm leaving the country. And then wonders why. Acts concerned. Wants to know more. That's the dream. That she still cares enough to ask why. To reach out. Unrealistic. This croissant is tainted because I bought it.

*

I watch a film on the flight over called *Me and Earl and the Dying Girl*. I'm sobbing so much I have to catch my breath. Could be the altitude. Could be my attitude. The positioning of my axis. Idle chat with the man across from me. I like being in business because I feel like I shouldn't be here. This guy's body language suggests he's here a lot. I play confident for a bit. Impress him. Move on.

Why do I feel like I shouldn't be in business? That's black-boy business. Brown-boy energy. Tricks of the system. The club lounge is a far cry from Neasden. Whenever I achieve a milestone in my life, Jake always says to me, 'Look at this! Little you from Neasden!'

Right now he'd say, 'Little you from Neasden flying business class!'

Even if I did hustle it. Right now isn't the best example. But the feeling is the same. When I'm here, feels like I've defied odds. Can't say my mum didn't show me the ropes. Broaden my horizons. She made me feel like the world was my oyster even when I bunked the train. I wanted to be a footballer back then. Like every single boy on my estate. If I hadn't made it in music, I would have kicked myself. My last real job was working in the fast-food section of a greyhound stadium. Used to come home smelling of oil.

And now look at me with my frizzy fucking hair and camo tracksuit. All up in your fucking business class. Yeah, give me that free shit (it's not even free). Yeah, let me put my feet up. Not a slave any more.

I am though. Because these thoughts'll plague me. They're abnormal. Freedom is the absence of want. 'Want' is a chain in itself. Some people grow up without the dream of buying their mum a house. Unreal.

The flight is long and I'm out of touch. I love that

phones don't work in the sky. My mind wanders. Pleasant daydreams and idyllic outcomes circle my head. Like a concussed cartoon character. Only for me to turn my phone on when I land. And have no messages from Chloe. Just one message from my phone network telling me that I've been charged twelve pounds in the first five minutes I've been here.

17

Can't Escape Yourself

'Remember that you're not a bad person.'
That's one of the last things a friend said to me before I left. After telling me I couldn't go to this party. Said sorry but it'd be unfair of him. Chloe didn't want to see me. Still. After about a month. I was hoping my invite would slip under the radar. So she could see me, unprepared. Face the reality. Look me in my eyes.

I'm not a good person. I know I'm not a good person. That's how I feel.

There's no room for nuance with cheating. Seems settled. Cheaters are bad people. Once a cheat always a cheat. Shit like that. Sickening. I felt sick all the time. The night before I left, I lay there in my bed. Scrolling Google search results. Blue light reflecting off glazed pupils. Aching for redemption. Kindness. Everything I read online was so aggressive. Full of rage. Black and white. I just wanted to read a post saying that there was a way back. That it was retrievable. Instead there were blog posts with lines like IF YOU'VE JUST CHEATED ON SOMEONE YOU LOVE, CONGRATULATIONS. YOU'VE JUST RUINED THEIR LIFE.

People who cheat are selfish and self-centred and deserve nothing.

It's not possible to cheat on someone you love. If you did, you never loved them.

I'd hear that a lot, actually. Maybe you didn't really love her. Is it that simple? You don't cheat on someone if you love them? Why do I care so much then? Why can't I seem to go a single waking minute without wishing I was asleep?

And all of us cheaters live under this big, itchy blanket. Woodlice that we are. No further interrogation. Someone is either a cheat or not a cheat. Right now, I'm covered in the same material as a man who fucked his ex behind his girlfriend's back for six months. Or a married man shagging his colleague on business trips. Or a woman sleeping with her husband's brother. Haven't heard much about women cheating. I've only really heard about men. But to quote my female friend: 'When women cheat, no one finds out.'

So it's a man thing, right now. That boy shit. Boys always want more. Boys always want to have their cake and eat it. Boys can't keep it in their pants. It's no surprise really. Boys will be boys. I didn't even have sex with the woman at the wedding. Now there's a hole inside me. Now I'm in the same sperm-filled ballpark as those who have premeditated their betrayal. I'm knocking about with repeat offenders. I fucked up once and then was honest about it. Still going to hell, it seems.

'You did the right thing.'

I get told that more often than not. The brave thing. Did I? Others say it's selfish. Only point is to relieve myself of guilt. That's why people are honest. To make themselves feel better. Isn't that the point? Otherwise it'll come out in other ways. Worm its way into conversation. Life'll become a collection of heart drops. Minor panics. Flipouts. It rots away at you, surely? And the regret becomes a permanent balaclava. You can no longer sit alone. Because when you do, you wonder where the other version of you would be. The one that owns up to their shit. It becomes a game. And, brutally, life is a game. Why's it even called 'cheating'?

Maybe I was relieving myself by being honest. In school I used to play this game called 'the game'. The only rule of the game was to not think about the game. Right now, I'm losing the game, for example. Every now and again somebody would announce that they'd lost the game and, in doing so, ruin everyone else's. You can't be winning the game unless you know you're playing. And there's no way of discovering if someone has never lost the game since finding out about it because you can't ask them.

That's how I used to respond to something like betrayal. Bury it so deep it feels forgotten. Morph a lie into reality. And the guilt felt when remembering was the eternal price you paid. For fucking up in the first place. Feeling awful was the consequence. And if there came a time when you remembered what had happened and didn't feel bad, you had lost more than the game. That's what I'd tell myself. The pain was because you care.

Shouldn't have done it in the first place.

That's another one I hear a lot.

Should have thought about it before you did it.

I find one website that claims to have particular methods

that may help get back a betrayed partner. No contact for sixty days was the first requirement. Already fucked that up.

*

My uncle's like something out of a Richard Curtis film. He's my mum's half-brother. Very British but now fully Brazilian. Forever in and out of love. When I arrive at his, he's sat topless at his kitchen counter. The light above him harsh and orange. Flies trying to kill themselves. He's happy to see me. Crow's feet and Brazilian Portuguese. Another melodic language. With passion and emphasis. We feel far from British monotony. Something he left thirty years ago. Three hundred quid and a briefcase. Built a life for himself. Brick by brick. Last time I visited him I was 15. With my mum. I remember the rain being warm. And him wanting me to taste the local rum. He was in a different home then. Had a different life. But he's still in Rio. More children and more passion. You can see the love in his eyes. He's almost worn out by it.

He knows I need to escape. But I was brief on the phone. He was excited to see me either way. Family and all that. I tell him that I cheated on my girlfriend and desperately want her back. His eyes are calm and compassionate. I feel like I've been chopped in half and he's counting the rings. Finding some kind of solace in remembering a time when heartbreak was new. He advises me to stay calm. Offers me a beer. I tell him I'm not drinking.

In the living room there's a photograph of a boy chasing his own shadow. I'm staying in the room of my little half-

half-cousins. I don't know how it works. We're related. They're not here at the moment. They're caught between a love that never lasted. So I'm on the bottom bunk of a bunk bed in a room with one window. The window is fenced from the outside. The neighbours are noisy. It's a boutique prison. Yoga mat on the floor. I'll probably do press-ups.

I want to join in with the noise outside but I can't. Pots, pans, cans and envy. My envy because I don't know how to be there. My uncle is in bed early because he wakes up at the crack of dawn. There will be mornings where we greet each other. I plan on doing therapy as much as possible but it'll be early morning to make the times work with the UK. I guess we'll wake up and share coffee. Which is on tap. I imagine I will struggle to stop drinking it.

18

Shock Resistance

I've been here a week now. Every morning I walk up to the nearest café and have a bowl of açai for breakfast. I fucking love açai. It was one of the parts of coming to Rio I was most looking forward to. This purple fruit. In the UK we use syrup to make it. In Rio there are cafés that have the real shit. Go in and everyone's mouths are purple. Lips, teeth, everything. Unapologetically.

I ring Tai, Jake and two or three other people in cycles throughout the day. I live for these phone calls. Updates. The feeling as though people care. In every conversation I'm searching for relief. A dove. Some rope. Reasons why I don't need to care about Chloe. Something that indicates Chloe might still be interested. Or my friends make jokes instead, and I get to throw my shit out the window for a second. But it always comes back. Boomerang that it is. I crave existential chat. Where I get to feel tiny, small and insignificant. Crave stuff about the state of the world. The delusion of the people. Ridiculous concepts. Human idiocy. I want to be a grain of sand on a beach of idiocy. I am. But it's easy to forget when I'm revolving around myself at such speed. Most of the time I just close my eyes so I don't get motion sickness.

One of my survival techniques is writing. It's always been an escape. A channel for anger. First time I wrote a rap was to diss my form tutor in school. Right now I'm struggling to find the words. Simple sentences hurt the most though. The final letter Chloe sent me was really fucking short. I run to the beach. I film myself running. Sun in the background. Proper desktop wallpaper stuff. I wish I felt like what I was running through. It's more of an eclipse for me. I stop running. I cry. I take a picture of myself crying. That's a new one. What does that mean? I don't post it anywhere. Am I planning to post it? Do I want people to know I'm sad? Do I want Chloe to know I'm sad? It's uncomfortable. Because I am authentically sad. And yet took a selfie. I'm sad OSX. I'm sad 8 Pro Max. But also – it's important to document. For so long I wasn't sad. Hid from it. Maybe a part of me doesn't want to let it go. I'm reading a book called *Dark Night of the Soul*. It stuck out to me in my uncle's bookcase. That and *The Happy Prince* by Oscar Wilde. It's about somebody who became so sad that they in turn freed themselves from emotional tyranny and became enlightened. Or something like that. This is my dark night of the soul.

Online. There's a hashtag #MeToo. It's wildfire. Countless accounts of men being abusive. Great time to have been cheated on, to be honest. From a woman's perspective. Men are trash. Put men in the bin. I've seen decent men aligning themselves with the cause. The movement feels right. Long overdue. My ex first became aware of me because I had written a poem about the interpersonal inequality that women face. Very ironic. Now I find parallels between myself and some of these antagonists. I've always been good at pointing the finger at everyone other than myself. Perhaps the fact I'd been honest would count for something. I'm certainly facing my own truth. I'm angry with her too, but there's no space for it.

It's all accountability right now. It's all shock resistance. I can't believe that I've never been taught how to not hurt myself. So I write. I write about the void I've found myself in. In between crying. In between cigarettes. Maybe other men lack a compass. Maybe they were never given one.

I can't believe no one warned me about heartbreak.

19

The Body Never Lies

It's all about my body. Our bodies. An undeniable differ-ence. Men got short-term strength. Quick power. Big bodies. An ex-girlfriend once said to me, 'You don't know what it's like to feel physically threatened during sex.'

And she was right. I've never feared for my life in that moment. Truly, anyway. Generally we have the bigger bodies. Strength. Power. But some of us lack responsibility. Why do we not feel proud of our bodies? Aware of our strength. To lift. We can lift so much if you want. Everything but ourselves. Out here fighting everything other than our demons.

I've spent years outside my body. Couldn't even feel my toes. It's difficult to know if men love their bodies. The sculpted ones. I see them. In the gym. On the screen. But they can be the worst. Obsessive. Insatiable. Uncomfortable. Overcompensating for a lack of direction. Yes, being healthy. Yes, we all need to feel strong. We need to. We should love our bodies and build muscle. But anything is toxic when taken to an extreme. There's a dysmorphia there. We wanna be like gods. Marvel gods. Like the films. Veins popping. Big, bulky. We're shown this unrealistic image. Fed chiseled abs. And the seed is supported. Sprouted. With shots of blushing women. Diet Coke with lemon. Magic Mike. Not all women. Men have space to relax at a certain age. Dad bods – they're sexy. And you can lose it if you want. No need to feel ashamed.

But I wonder about the shame of our bodies. I argued with a man once. I had suggested that 'everyone was bisexual' during a group discussion. Yes, it was a large comment. Vast. Provocative, maybe. He said, 'If you're coming out, mate, just say so. Don't try and tell me what I like.'

I told him that I wasn't coming out. I was suggesting that for men it would be difficult to know, being that we so heavily shame male intimacy. Why can women fuck around with each other when they're young and still be straight? Two straight women can kiss for men's enjoyment and that's not seen as 'gay'?

I spoke of these double standards. The conversation continued. I made the point about straight women doing gay porn. I interrogated the notion of what homophobic even means. It got to the point where the man said, 'I love watching women have sex because I find women so attractive. I don't even find men 1 per cent attractive.'

Imagine not being able to find men attractive. How do you know if you yourself are attractive?

It's anything to not feel shame. That's the energy. Avoidance. And the worst shame comes from something we can't change. Perpetuated by nearly everyone. Dick size. Weaponised. Nonsensical parallels. Between behaviour and genitalia. Doesn't even make sense. And height. Ridiculous. What happens to the men who can't escape? Feel small? Does it mutate?

I don't like double standards.
They have no body to them.

*

My uncle is a man of faith. He practises an Afro-Brazilian religion called Candomblé. He wears white. Beads too. He is white. The faith is one of enslaved Africans but he breathes it. Somehow. In spite of the Hugh Grant look. His proximity has wandered. His current girlfriend is black. Absolutely gorgeous. Massive afro. He keeps suggesting I should come with him one afternoon. Speak to the priestess. I'm hesitant. I too am a person of faith but I don't know where to aim it. I just know that there's more going on. I believe it with my whole body. I've experienced it. I'm still a cynic though. Like I said. Pinch of salt. And if everyone's wearing white. I'm not sure. But I agree. At some point. I can tell that my uncle is a little concerned about me.

20

Fear

I've heard whispers that we don't know fear. That we're protected. Guarded. Unaware. Spinning around in meadows. Not true. Not all of us. Don't forget the incisions. Intersections. Violence has many forms. We all know fear. Different masks. Same tears.

You could say. You don't know fear until you claim to have no fear. The fear of not being fearless. A fear of leaning. Balancing on one foot. Breathing slowly. Fear got us by the neck. And we're frowning. Growling. Frothing at the fucking mouth. What if somebody finds out? What if those secrets come out? The ones trapped in our tendons. The hiccups. The slip-ups. Accidentally telling her the truth at five in the morning. Getting drunk and being honest. Getting high and being honest. She knows what I'm like naked. Dick out. Soft.

Don't be scared though. That's the message, right? Men aren't scared. Big boys aren't scared. Can't be scared of being poor. Losing opportunities. Falling down ladders. Can't be broke or broken. Sexual economy. What are you worth? What are dicks worth? Can't be scared of fighting. Protecting. Risking. Can't be scared of risk. No fear.

Fearless. Unless we're talking femininity. Now we're scared. Scared of being seen as feminine. Fearless but also homophobic? Somehow. Scared of homosexuality. Something human since the dawn of time. Natural like the sunrise. Fearless though. Can't be scared of putting on weight. Not having abs. Hairline going. Teeth fucked. Can't be scared of carbs. Or the silence of sobriety. No, can't be scared of drinking. Blacking out. Regret.

Can't be scared of rejection. Abandonment. Have a lover crush your heart like orange juice. Duck out. Cut out. Can't be scared of love. Diversion tactics. Can't be losing control. So we don't need it. We don't need love. What's the point if it hurts? Emotional pain hits different. Hits too hard.

But all men know if you get hit too hard, you must be stone. Never let the blood run out. Someone might see. No one can see the blood. People get protective over things they care about. People put their guard up. Out of fear. How then can our hearts be considered stone? Perhaps they in fact feel so much that our teeth sharpen.

21

Touched by the Other Side

We're in a taxi driving out of the city in Rio, my uncle and me. Industrial, grey buildings. Cracks. Lines. Curves. It's the grey that grabs you though. And the closeness. Taxi tyres kicking up filth. Wide highway. We're moving away from the heartbeat – or towards it. It's all based on perspective. There are mountains above the grey. Blue sky above the grey. Colourful clothes hang and speckle the grey, but it still feels solid. A doorstop. That people live in.

My uncle tells me that no one at his place of faith speaks English. He'll have to translate. Assures me. Soothes me. Explains to me why he only speaks to his dog in Arabic. Feels rural now. Car takes a corner. Heads up a half-finished street. Craters and holes. Injuries. Some decent bungalows. Sparse. Beware of the dogs. Cacti. No one to be seen yet. Cars need dusting. Taxi stops and the heat kicks in. Air is heavy. Sun is high. We approach the house.

White everything. Walls, gate and clothing. My uncle dialogues with a couple of people straight away. Shakes hands, introduces me. We walk into the house. My uncle turns to me and says, 'If you feel the urge to sleep, go in there.'

Points to a room of two bunk beds. Already a couple of people out cold. He continues: 'That's how the orishas get to work here. Through rest. Make sure you welcome it.'

Orisha meaning god. Walk into the kitchen. Grandma type by the stove. Stirring a pot. Summer dress, glasses. Calm but guarded. Portuguese exchange. Uncle fluent. In movement too. Dances into the backyard. A few others sit at a table. Loose fabric mimics the tongue. Plastic bowls of goodness on the table. Hand gesture to sit down. Welcoming. My uncle tells me that we eat and sweep.

The food's good. More people arrive. Seems as though there's an event. More Portuguese and wonder grins. I try and stay close to my uncle for ease but don't want to be too clingy. In the moments when I can't see him I check my phone. In a perpetual state of expectation. A reassuring text. There's one other person who speaks a little English. A kind man who looks like a boy. Big eyes. Suggestion of a moustache. He lives around here, out of the city. Dusty trainers. There's not much around here from what I can see. Places like this used to freak me out as a kid. Having been raised in the city, I couldn't understand how people could live so far from sport shops. How would they be able to look at football boots? I'd also consider how long it would be after you died that anyone would realise. I realise these thoughts were irrational. Still, it's always been stillness that rattles me. Any space too tranquil, I don't know what to do with it. Things have to be moving, surely? I wish my heart was still. I'm starting to understand how important it is to stop.

Plus I could imagine myself now, standing on one of these corners, with a lemonade, watching the world go by.

I'm handed some white robes and trousers. I can be part of the experience now. There's some special water in a bucket. I'm to wash myself in it. And stick the clothes on. All part of the ceremony. There's an outhouse in the back garden. I notice people come in and out of it as they sweep. I ask my uncle to take me in. Inside there's a huge altar. Candles, photographs, drawings. All in appreciation of one particular orisha. Offerings. It's powerful. I feel it in my chest. Still, I don't know what anyone's saying and feel disorientated. My uncle gives me a smile. Big one. I nod. Next, people gather in a circle.

Music is playing and people are swaying. I'm on the outside looking in. Wanting and trying to appreciate. Suddenly my uncle becomes possessed. He begins moving in a childlike fashion with his hands covering his eyes. Sometimes flat against his face. Sometimes facing outwards like *Pan's Labrinth*. He's stomping, making noises, giggling. Everyone's vibing with it. My Britishness kicks in. I hold back from frowning. From thinking this is all a bit embarrassing. At least a fifth of me is cynical. I have to provide balance to my dreaminess. Everyone seems cool with this though. Now he's grunting and stamping his foot. Another person joins in. I keep wondering why it's my uncle who's going through this while I'm here. I don't know if that's usual or not. Is he doing this in front of me to prove a point? I keep my eyes on the mother of the household. The grandma type from earlier. She appears to be the matriarch here. She's vibing. Must be all good. Time passes and it's over. My uncle opens his eyes. Big smile again. Seems a little wired. Acknowledges me briefly. Then we all wind down.

I ask him what just happened. He says he was channelling one of the orishas who often comes through the earth in the back garden. I nod as if I understand. He tells me that later on I can have my runes read by the grandmother. Says it's one of the oldest religious practices on earth. She sits in front of you and throws a handful of cowry shells. Those beautiful shells you always see on necklaces or interwoven into locks. The shells indicate which orisha is watching over you. Sometimes it's more than one.

Before this I have to take a sacred shower in the specially prepared water. I've got to lift a bucket over my head and bathe myself in it. The showers are outside. Little cubicles. I go into one. Remove my clothing. Have my new white outfit ready. I bathe myself in the sacred water. I can then turn on the actual shower and bathe myself some more if I'd like. After I do, there's a moment – very short. A short, inexplicable moment. Can't believe it. Stood still for a moment afterwards while my mind rejigged and the water fell on me. Trickled down me. I was overcome. Possessed. I snorted out through my nose. Dragged back a single foot and stamped on the ground. Like an animal. Like the orisha that was being channelled earlier. As if. I battle with the notion that I've just been inhabited by an energy.

I don't mention anything to my uncle. I keep it moving. I'm overwhelmed. I'm thinking about my phone which is on charge in the other room. Unsure of what I just experienced. I'm about to have my runes read. We walk into the shed which has the altar inside. The grandmother is sat at a small table. She's been guiding others. We sit. They speak. My uncle translates.

The shells are beautiful. The sun beams through the

shed window. The grandmother is sturdy. No need to please. Little grin to help settle. The runes are thrown. She begins to analyse. Vocalising what she can see and feel. My uncle is taking it all in. I look at him nervously. I have no idea what's coming. Can't gauge where she's at either.

My uncle begins to translate. 'She says that you have two orishas guiding you. They're both here now. But there is some kind of conflict . . .'

'Eh? What do you mean?'

'She's saying that the orishas are opposed to each other. One of them is a god of time and wind. The other is a god of war.'

'Oh, right. Woah.'

'They are two very powerful orishas. But she says that you are currently at a crossroads and you have to ensure that you are balanced enough to move in a positive direction . . . She says that in all the twenty-two years she's been practising she's never met a single person that's guided by these two orishas at the same time.'

'What? Is that special then? A good thing?'

My uncle pauses a little while she speaks some more. He talks back. I feel as though none of this is real. Twenty-two years, he just said. Never in all her time practising. Am I supposed to feel special? This feels like one of those moments. I used to have them when I was a kid. Is this proof that I am some kind of chosen one? Is everything fantastic in the world going to happen to me? Am I mortal? If I walk out onto the highway, will I actually die?

'Yes, it is a powerful thing. But you must treat the situation with care.'

'Ok.'

'She's suggesting you come back here for a spiritual intervention.'

'An intervention?'

'I think you should do it. We can discuss later.'

I'm baffled. Attention back to grandmother. She's more open now. Smiling a little more. She mutters to my uncle. He says she's asking me if there's anything else at all I want to ask the orishas while I'm here. Anything. I look at my uncle first. Search his face for signs of safety. I ask him if it's inappropriate to ask them about this breakup specifically. About heartbreak. He bends his lips and shakes his head. Not at all. I say ok then. Ask her to ask them about that. He does. She nods. Waits a moment. Replies.

My uncle translates. 'She says that this person you've broken up with has no interest in repairing things. You're better off moving on.'

Didn't want to hear that.

22

'Too Depressed for Eastern Medicine'

I'm on a dating app. A special one. One for people with followings. You know the one. Celebrities, models, footballers. Occasionally a photographer with no fucking following at all. Must be mates with one of the owners. It's pretty vacuous. But exciting. I feel special being on it, getting to see who else is single. I want to match with everyone. Especially the women with editorial fashion shoots. Anything for a lift. I haven't had much come from it. Chloe told me once that she saw me on there before but didn't match me 'cause her friend wanted to instead. Good times. Internet dating is so wild. Surely attraction is based off energy. Real-life energy. Not PowerPoint presentations. Still, the validation is addictive. Watching slideshows. Imagining what life could be like. Pure fantasy. I know one guy who married a woman off this app. I've seen a picture and she's stunning. My friend, Ruthy, who knows them said it's an awful relationship and she's a fucking nightmare.

When I show my uncle a picture of Chloe he droops. A memory from his own past tumbles off him. He nods ever so slightly, pushes out a little breath. We both sip our black filtered coffee. He says that beauty's not always a good thing. Aesthetic beauty anyway. It comes with its own challenges. Ultimately it's the content of someone's character that shines through. And he thinks she looks sad in the picture I showed him. Not the first time someone's said that. It's a picture from a great day, genuinely.

My uncle suggests I get acupuncture. Says he's got a mate. One of the best in Rio – of course. Says he can fit me in, will sort me out. I thank him and leave to get an açai bowl.

*

Another perk of reasonable success. Being able to afford therapy. It shouldn't be so expensive but it is. I'm having therapy three times a week while I'm out here. On Skype. At peculiar hours because of the time difference. Sometimes I'm already just lying in my bed awake. My therapist is keen to break through with me. If it's triple therapy I need then it's what I need. And I'm wide open. I am a gaping wound. My therapist wants me to acknowledge my core emotions. Not my inhibitory ones. She uses a form of therapy called IEDP. It's fascinating. It's not at all like the therapy I've seen on screen. Or heard about. It's not talk therapy. I talk to her of course, but she's paying attention to how I'm saying things. Watching my body. Studying my cadence. According to this method of therapy, anxiety and depression are not in themselves emotions. They're actually our body preventing us from feeling our core emotions. A defensive strategy. Survival shit learnt when we're young. I'd never looked at it like this. But it makes sense. She tells me about something called the Change Triangle. An interpretation of IEDP coined by a woman called Hilary Jacobs Hendel, who talks a lot about male trauma specifically and seems especially attuned to those specific challenges. And my therapist is still watching me. My eyes. Encouraging me to verbally acknowledge emotions. Map the journey towards them. I am yawning because I am anxious. I am anxious because I am sad and my body is trying to control it. Say that you are sad. Out loud. Say that you are angry. Apparently consciously acknowledging these emotions begins processing them. Otherwise they get lodged. I ran up a set of stairs the other day and burst into tears. My therapist wants me to talk more about my mum. She wonders if I actually view her as my mum.

She notes moments when I'm defensive. When I guard myself from harmless enquiries. As if I'm being judged. My therapist wonders why I feel like she's judging me. She was disappointed I never told her about cheating. She feels she could have helped the situation play out in a more balanced way. She's not wrong. These sessions are the nearest thing I have to a womb right now. Would love to crawl back inside a womb. I feel regret. A lot. But the idea is for me to be compassionate to myself. To understand why I acted in that way. To know that those actions came from pain. And that that side of me deserves love too. My love. For sure. Yes, I'm trying not to punish myself. But it's all I know. It's something I observed a lot as a child. My mum has always been very hard on herself.

*

My dreams have been a world of fear and safety. Some mornings I wake up and my chest tightens immediately. And I wish I was asleep again. In a different world. Where I don't feel like this. Even if it was a nightmare, I'd almost rather be there.

I used to have nightmares a lot as a child – at times almost every night. I'd be stuck in horrific situations and the only way I could escape was by dying. I had to die every night to wake up. No wonder I had such a sweet disposition. I was over the moon every morning. Having just been stabbed to death or burned alive. My most vivid nightmare was of me and my mum. Both of us would be sat in the flat's living room. Doing something. Playing chess. Everything as normal. Purple and orange walls. Material hung like a painting. And then the room would break into two. My universe would rupture. On the other side was my mum. Floating further and further away, into the stars. Galaxies and black holes. They were my favourite thing to read about as a kid. Stars. Solar systems. And now my mum was disappearing into them. And I was on the other side holding my hands out. Wondering whether or not I could make the jump.

*

I can't find the acupuncturist for a while. The pin is taking me in and out of this Brazilian mall. Fuckin' annoying, and it's fuckin' hot. I text my uncle asking for the guy's number. Flick through that fucking dating app. Don't match anyone. Number comes through. I ring him. Find the door. It is a bit hidden, to be fair. Press the buzzer and I'm up.

He seems chill. Completely what I'd expect an acupuncturist to look like. And sound like. He invites me to sit in front of him. The other side of his desk. We exchange politeness, then he asks me to stick my tongue out. I do. Then he says, 'You have an issue with anger.'

I retract my tongue. Who fucking doesn't? How the fuck does he know? From my tongue. It's all my therapist has been saying. Says it's the root of my addiction – potentially. Fury. All stuffed in my solar plexus. Taken out of myself. Theory is: as a child I was angry. Fuming in fact. With my parents. At times. For not looking after me in the way I needed. For various reasons. We were poor, stressed, distracted. And my parents were superheroes in my eyes. Especially as an only child. But I became aware, too young perhaps, that things were difficult. And so shielded them from my anger. In the hope it would make things ok. Didn't want to be the final Jenga block. But anger needs to move. Otherwise it becomes corrosive. So I learnt to take it out on myself. Or try to escape the feeling of it being there. Now it's all over my fucking tongue.

The acupuncturist then directs me towards the table in the middle of the room. Palm out, open. Kind. I remove a few items of clothing and lay down. He gets together his little pack of needles. Sits down by my feet and gets going. I'm ok with needles. More so when they're bigger. Little ones freak me out. Remind me of *Hellraiser*. I worry about rolling over. Pin prick. Nerve twitch. Blood shift. He talks it through with me. The process. The journey. At some point, he asks me about mindfulness. Pulls out a little device. Something I can clip on my finger. Says it measures the meditative state of his clients. Lets him know if they've entered a full state of relaxation. That way the whole process has another level. It's a technique he's added to the practice. He asks me to shut my eyes and go to my 'happy place'. To visit a memory that brings me joy. I close my eyes and see nothing. I feel clogged. Hair in a drain. Honestly, nothing. I'm laying horizontally and gravity is on my face. On my neck. Heavier than normal. Adam's apple like an asteroid. I'm magnetically attached to the centre of the earth right now. Didn't know you could choke on nothing. He looks at the device. Says I'm not quite getting there.

'Just think of a happy memory,' he says again. As if I haven't fucking tried to. My eyes have an inch of water balancing on top of them, being that I'm facing the ceiling. Salt streams rolling down each cheek. Throat sealed shut. I start asking myself why I can't see anything. Why can't I see anything happy? Which makes everything feel even more severe. The tie feels tighter. The acupuncturist even gets frustrated. He might as well jump on the table and scream, 'Why aren't you happy?' while facing down on me like a scene from a Hollywood gangster film. I don't know. I'm sure frustration is inappropriate in this environment. While I have grief on my face. Like a wet flannel. He just wants me to be mindful. I want to be mindful too. What bliss that would be. I would love to be in a happy place right now. I would love to return to a single joyous memory. And they exist, by the way. Of course they exist. I've got drawers full of fun times. I just can't get them open. Something's stuck. And the sound of the drawer's lock crashing against the inside of the cabinet is giving me anxiety.

Eventually he gives up. I cause him to put down the mindfulness finger device. He seems almost deflated. As if I've popped this acupuncturist's balloon.

He composes himself and we return to his desk. He waits a couple of beats and then says that I am in fact a lot sadder than he could have ever predicted. In a very kind way he continues by saying that my heart is truly broken and he suggests I take it easy. The words bounce off my face. I say thank you, leave and stride into humid Brazilian air. I plan on having an açai bowl in a lovely café. Somewhere I can process what just happened.

*

I walk my uncle's dog. The one he shouts at in Arabic. She's pretty chill. Pocket rocket. She can walk off the lead which is cool. I would only ever want a dog I can walk off the lead. We've got a little routine going. Our own route. I walk past the houses of people I will never know having conversations I will never understand. The houses are all much more vibrant than in England. Just the choice of colour. Pastel peaches and pinks. Or perhaps the sun just makes everything look better. I wish I had this weather all year, I really do. Historically I've had girlfriends who have all expressed a love for winter. They're always talking to me about jumpers and hot chocolates and shit. But I just objectively enjoy light. I love the day. There's definitely something comforting about snuggling under a blanket and creating your own warmth. But then there's having that snuggle from the actual sun itself. Even the winter sun is my favourite part of winter. Maybe I've got to improve my relationship with darkness. I am chasing my shadow at the moment, after all.

The dog is called Luna. I've honestly never met so many dogs called Luna. I wonder what it is about that name. My favourite dog names are the most human ones. Like Susan. Or Sandra. Or Nathan. Or Jerome. At one point Luna goes off a little further to sniff a pack of dogs up the road. The dogs are all on leads being held by a disgruntled-looking short woman with a hat on. As Luna gets near she pulls out a taser and clicks it in Luna's direction. I'm in shock. Luna evades her. Probably thinks 'fuck that'. I move towards Luna and put her on the lead. The dog walker walks past me. I ask her why the fuck she just did that. She doesn't even register me being there. Not one bit.

The acupuncturist texts my uncle. He tells him that I'm 'too depressed for Eastern medicine'. And that I should consider antidepressants or a spiritual intervention of some kind. My uncle tells me this but doesn't stand by it necessarily. He's drawn to the suggestion of a spiritual intervention, given that this had already been suggested at the Candomblé house. Also, the grandmother has offered to move other ceremonies in order to facilitate me before I leave. Which is a massive honour, according to my uncle. I believe him. I agree to do it.

23

When One Door Closes

It always seems to be father this, father that. His father is farther away, that's why. Distant father. Oh no, poor him. Poor statistic. Poor probability. That's what it is, you know. It's the lack of a father figure. Yes. I would agree, actually. Fathers do disappear. And we get stuck in a loop. A cycle. How to father with no father. But it's not always, always, always that. Trust. The mums too. Listen. There are more than a few superheroes out there. Mothers who lift cars, buses. But it's not all roses. Mother son, mother son, mother son. It's not always plain sailing. Less obvious. Hidden round the corner. What happens if she doesn't let go? Psyches him out. What happens if she sees his dad in him. Does she take it out on him? Is he a reminder? Does he get punished? What happens if he falls in love and his attention is drawn to another woman? Is it always a walk in the park? I know boys teased by their mums. Beaten by their mums. Degraded by their mums. I know boys obsessed with their mums. Do anything for their mums. Leave anyone for their mums. The mother close to the son. It can get tricky. Because it's often undetected. Encouraged. Celebrated. Look how lovely he is with his mum. Has he left her womb though? Does he want to get back in? I know I do sometimes. Is that weird?

*

My uncle's girlfriend is beautiful. And she has a sister who is beautiful too. The sister is visiting her at the moment. Adds to the vibe. My uncle arranges a dinner up in the mountains. Impeccable skin. His girlfrend opens her mouth when she smiles. She's not that much older than me. Don't know if that's weird or not. They have a clear energy between them. It feels orderly and driven. Muscly. She has eyes that ask questions. Not instantly accessible like me. I find myself wide open very quickly. Trusting. Believing. I feel like she's prepared to say no. Her sister is older than her. Similar qualities except the accentuation is in her cheeks. Whereas with my uncle's girlfriend it's more in the jaw. Her older sister's eyes are a little bigger. She's a little taller. And her big afro kind of flops down on either side. Her English is also a lot better.

Up in the mountains everything is romantic. People with faces like peach pits. Full of stories. No doubt my uncle's booked a good spot. We walk in a golden sheen. Homely but clean. Polished. We all take our seats, but not long after we do I excuse myself. I walk outside and ring Tai. For the second time today. And I reel while treading dust. Trying not to be too loud. More of the same. Chloe has maintained contact with him, which feels cruel. But I'm trying to decipher everything she says and does. Tai suggests he stops speaking to her. But I say no. It's still contact. It's still something. Don't let go.

But the more we talk, the more I hear myself. And I find myself at a bridge. The middle of the bridge overlooks the middle of Rio. I'm up a fucking mountain. And it's so quiet. I've walked far enough from the restaurant now. Maybe this is residential. I'm not on the phone any more. My ear feels hot from pushing the phone so close to my face. It's so quiet, and then my head isn't. Voices appear.

A friend once told me about 'the imp of the perverse'. A definition online defines it as 'a metaphor for the urge to do exactly the wrong thing in a given situation for the sole reason that it is possible for wrong to be done'. Based on an essay by Edgar Allan Poe. I've always had the voice. Whenever I'm on a platform. On a balcony. In a car on the motorway. I get this overbearing urge to jump. Leap. Open the door. Fantasising about how simple it would be. And what a relief. But I'm always fighting it and I never do. And I was having those thoughts before I was heartbroken. Wasn't even in pain really. And now I fucking am. And I'm on this bridge looking down. And thinking of the peace. The eternal sleep. No more barbed-wire breathing. No more wet cheeks. If I just stepped off, walked on air. Word is that you pass out from the shock before you hit the ground. Is that peaceful? What if you don't pass out? Is it selfish? It's difficult to see more than a foot ahead of me. What happens when it's done? I'm not going to jump right now. No. Doesn't feel right.

We sit and eat. My uncle's girlfriend is called Elissa. Her sister is called Shamica. Shamica is sat to the left of me. The food is great, conversation fluid. Hard not to feel like it's a bit of a double date. I mask my sorrow with comedy. Make jokes. I make Shamica laugh. Giggle even. And she shifts her body towards me a little. Just re-angles ever so slightly. Conversation moves on to her husband. It seems polite. I feel a different energy from her though. In a different dimension I flirt. What a taboo. Proper rush. But I just don't have the energy. My uncle mentions that I'm heartbroken. She responds with a sigh. Tilt of the head. Says she's going to a party later and I can come if I fancy.

We leave the mountains. I hear a wolf howling. I imagine a wolf howling. I'm back in my prison room. Thinking about that party. About drinking. So many variables. Fantasies about Shamica. Reviewing my guesses that she's unhappy in her relationship. Measuring the damage of a beer. I can hear parties, gatherings, through the bars in the window. Noise. But all I want is updates. Thumbing down my phone screen. A *Black Mirror* murder scene. Prints everywhere. Comfort. Reassurance. Distraction. I struggle to even watch shows or films because characters will remind me of her. Or stories graze the surface. The stones skim. And I skim-read articles. Wince at self-help. Attach myself to intellectual freedoms. I like hearing about friends' issues too. Feeling like I'm helpful. Rejigging my desperation. But too often I give people advice that I don't take myself and am left wondering why. Why, if I know objectively what the right steps are, can I not take them? Because pain doesn't make sense. It doesn't listen to answers. It just exists. In lakes and rivers beneath my organs. They say that when one door closes, another one opens. And it's always hopeful. But what if the door that opens leads to utter hell? What if the door that closed was to an infinite meadow of joy?

*

My therapist says that smoking is a 'defence', which is a reaction to an 'inhibitory emotion', in this case anxiety, which prevents me from experiencing a core emotion like anger. The Change Triangle. I tell her I feel guilt. I feel incredibly guilty. She says guilt is more complex. It's not a core emotion but it's not invalid. Guilt helps us gauge where we are. Or how we feel. Or if we care. But it shouldn't linger. Otherwise it turns into punishment. Self-harm. She knows this of me. She says it's good to feel regret but an immediate sense of guilt shouldn't follow feeling angry. Grief is so confusing. I am punishing myself. And I feel angry. And I am punishing myself. Every day I'm writing letters. Plotting emails. Chloe has told me to stay away. Leave her alone. Not talk to her. And it's all I can think about. What if I say something that changes her mind?

I told the truth because I wanted to face my shadow self. And that came in the shape of her face becoming maddened. It's all I can see. The moment when it landed. Replaying in my head constantly. Just one sentence and everything changed. And I thought, it's not like I stabbed her. It's not physical pain. But actually it's like stabbing someone again and again and again. Psychological pain isn't easily mended. So, yes, I'm in a feedback loop. A never-ending rollercoaster. In and out of a haunted house.

Again and again. Hurting someone again and again. Causing pain. A pain giver.

How unforgivable.

24

Cutting Ties

Couple of days after the mountain dinner, I've decided to break up with my mum. I didn't realise the extent of our relationship till now. Here in Brazil. Because there's so much to appreciate. I have so much to give thanks for. It's been me and her against the world for a long time. Fighting the system, fighting schools and fighting each other. She's given everything to keep me alive. Maybe too much. Without my mum I wouldn't have had such blind belief in myself. I wouldn't have had the drive to sit in my room and focus on my future. To constantly stand back up after being punched or belittled by other kids my age. And in reverse. She'd back it. In football she'd be on the sidelines, often the only woman there, shouting at the referee. Backing me even if I'd flown in recklessly on someone. Which I often did. It's hard to come to terms with how I'm feeling. Because mums are so fucking special. And I can't understand why life isn't entirely orientated around birth. Around that sacred cycle. Where existence is created and nurtured. Housed. It's unfathomable. And a lot of us grow up in debt. An unpayable one. I have soundbites and clips in my head of boys with their mums. Of girls talking about boys with their mums. Women discussing men with their mums. Loving your mum is a good thing. Above everything else. I love my mum an awful lot. Painful amount. I'd give up everything for her. But the truth is I can't give her what I want to give her.

As far back as I can remember, when the song was sung and flames lit my face, I've blown out my birthday candles and wished for my mum to be happy. Imagined my wish snaking up to a higher power. And then waiting. Because I knew. Even with her encouragement and support and belief in me. Even with my *Sonic the Comic* subscription and our trips to buy football boots and the breakfasts and lunches and dinners and colours and music and mixtapes and sunglasses and bright lipstick, I could tell. I was more aware of how she treated herself than anything else. The words she'd say to herself. Fighting cigarettes. And desserts. The immovable desire to be independent. Strong in some senses. Sad in others. I want her to be hugged in a way I can't provide. Someone her size and wise. Part of me wonders if all my drive, ambition, creativity, spark, resilience and belief has been amplified in an attempt to find a destination where my mother smiles and hugs herself. All the encouragement, fantasy, wonderment, freedom and protection in the world couldn't change the reality that I could always tell how she was feeling. I could feel it in my own body.

My mum wasn't unhappy the whole time. But stress would overshadow her. I wonder if that's why we had so many lamps. Fairy lights. Candles. To push away the shadows. There was a lamp in my bedroom that would morph into all kinds of shapes in the night. I swear I could hear it growl. I wouldn't say I was ever afraid of the dark as a kid. I might have been afraid that there wouldn't be light again.

I write my mum a message. I say that we need to let each other go and that I need to stop giving her things. I need to stop putting myself second. I don't mean stop being loving or giving or any other quality she's instilled in me. But just not giving at the sole expense of myself. It's not sustainable. And the world is cruel. I need boundaries. I keep hearing that word being thrown around. I need to find a way to be free so that my mum and I can reform a mature bond as equals.

I send the message. Another heartbreak. I leave my phone. I walk outside. I sit on a bench in the middle of the street and cry. No one's about. Not that it matters. I don't even understand what people are saying around me. It's hot. There are trees either side of me. And I sob. And smoke. And sob. And smoke. And it goes so deep this time. I find this space somewhere on the other side of my tears where all my senses are heightened. I hear a car turning a corner up the road. Kids giggling in the distance. The tree above me hisses. Scratches at the air like white noise. Comforting. I wipe my eyes and look up. The sun is silhouetting the shapes of the leaves. And bouncing around the gaps to find me. I look back down and see the shadows dance. The sunbeams warming the stone, shifting its tone. I can fucking feel it all in the moment. I take a deep breath.

*

When I was 7 my after-school club in London entered a local talent competition. I decided I wanted to be SisQó. SisQó had silver hair. His album was called *Unleash The Dragon*. I wanted to unleash the dragon. My mum found silver hair spray. It turned my afro grey. We found a shirt with dragons on at the market. We dyed it green just like SisQó would. Every day I practised lip-synching to his chart smash 'Thong Song'.

Had no idea what a thong was. Just knew he wanted to see it. I thought he was the coolest motherfucker, I swear. There's a part at the end of the song where the beat drops down before building again. SisQó says, 'Yeah, come on,' five or six times, then eventually the synth reaches a crescendo and he fucking goes for it. This guy could really sing. He would let his soul come out his mouth. But I was only lip-synching. So I planned to go into a Bruce Lee stance during the build. Then perform a super high karate kick when it dropped to emphasise the athleticism of his singing.

Every day I would practise. Especially the kick. Got to the day of the show and I fucking shit myself. I had sunglasses too by this point, to complete the look. I was at the side off stage. My mum was filming me on her VHS camera. 'You can do it, honey!' That vibe. I was so nervous I started body popping. The act before me walked off stage triumphantly. Walking on there now seemed so insane. Like a truly unusual thing to do. I froze.

My mum put down the camera for a second, held me and said, 'I know it feels scary to walk on right now, but once you do, you won't want to come off. I promise you that.'

My name gets announced. She nudges me in the back. I walk on. I perform. Three and a half minutes later the curtains close. And I actually come back out from behind them and clap myself.

From then I was hooked. My mum knew I would be. And a lifetime of complexity was ushered in. Standing out. Being the centre of attention. Getting high off appreciation. It all started there. With the best intentions. And good has certainly come from it. I could do with clapping myself now though. I could do with that energy.

25

The Power

Yeah, I'm off social media. Unthinkable. Sometimes the most noticeable thing you can do is disappear. I wanted Chloe to feel me go. To wonder. Ask questions. Think of me. And more importantly I wanted to separate from the chaos. Oil and water. Social media is unforgiving to malleable states. But of course I search anyway. I look for her updates. When I shouldn't. And it feels like she's playing. Toying. Cat and mouse. Photo shoots in lingerie. All in. I'm-single-hit-me-up energy. Honey traps. No prisoners. And I die with every refresh. Every time the page loads I die. Hoping there hasn't been another upload. Before I tear myself away again. Re-engage with my stark reality. Call a friend to massage me through it. Some friends would enable bright outcomes. Conspire to believe that it's all in my favour. Somehow.

'Have you seen what she's uploaded on Instagram?' I'd say.

'Yeah, you talking about the sexy shoot?' they'd say.

'Yes. What do you think?'

There'd be a pause. Friends with heart in their palms. 'I think she misses you.'

'Really?'

'Yes, of course.'

'But I don't think she cares about me any more. Honestly. Why would she be putting all these photos up if she misses me? What if she's already sleeping with someone else? Should I be looking for someone else?'

'I think you should focus on feeling better and not rush into anything. It hasn't been that long.'

'Are you fucking kidding? It's been about five years . . .'

'It's been a couple months at a push . . .'

'Time is a fucking joke.'

'Do you really want her back? Have you really thought about it?'

'Yes, I've thought about it and I do want her back. Or at least just want her to talk to me. I don't think she misses me. She can't have even loved me, to be honest. It doesn't make any sense.'

'You're giving her an awful lot of power by feeling like this.'

'What do you mean?'

'You're making it out as if only she can make you feel better. More so than yourself. That's not right. How can she have that much power? You need to make yourself feel better.'

Tears. Smoke. Salt. Ash. Burning. Swimming. All of that.

'Why's she being so fucking horrible?' I'd say. I'd vent. I'd make it feel like I was the one being hurt now. Like I'm the one being stabbed.

I have most of my phone conversations in my uncle's car park. It's always full. It's not underground, it just sits at the bottom of the building. I look up and see plants and washing lines. Clothes. Rarely faces. I imagine what it'd be like, boiling the kettle and overhearing a foreign voice three times a day, every day, for more than a week. Shouting, screaming, crying. I'd think, 'Shit, they must be going through it,' then I'd finish making my peppermint tea. Squeeze in a bit of honey and carry on with my day.

*

Talking about power. My uncle tells me a story about a prisoner he filmed when making a documentary. That's what my uncle does. He runs a production company. This guy he was interviewing was serving four life sentences or something. He'd done wild shit. Awful, reprehensible shit. High-security prison. And the deepest part was he loved it. He would talk about how much he loved watching people's heads explode. He loved seeing life leave people's eyes. He showed no remorse. Basked in the malevolence. So, as part of this documentary, they allowed these prisoners to take part in a ceremony. A plant ceremony. Ayahuasca or something. Deep spiritual healing. This guy did it. This cold-blooded killer. And guess what happened?

He has a vision and sees one of his victims. One of the people he'd killed. That person walked right up to him and said, 'I forgive myself for being killed by you.'

Not 'I forgive you for killing me'.

The guy said, 'I forgive myself for being killed by you.'

Apparently the murderer came back around a changed man. Couldn't believe it. The exchange had totally removed his power from that situation. He realised that he lived within people's perception of him. People vilified him and he embodied it. Full-body villain. Revelled in being evil. But to have that mat pulled from under him. For a 'victim' of his to understand a power way beyond either of them. To acknowledge a karmic cycle that transcends personality. Was life-changing.

I hold on to that story in my mind. Think about how to get my power back. Think about whether or not Chloe forgives herself. I feel good for two hours then look on Chloe's Instagram.

*

There's a famously incorrect internet quotation attributed to Oscar Wilde, 'Everything in the world is about sex, except sex. Sex is about power.'

And so I think about power and what I deem as powerful while I'm sat in this bunk bed. Am I the powerful one? Am I the dangerous, damaging one? Am I the problem? I look on the computer. Web full of fury. Stories of men. Male bullshit. Men are trash. Abuse of power. Sex is an arena where power has confused me. Escaped me. In my early teen years, 12, 13, girls felt monstrous. Towering. Horny. Seriously. The 12-year-old girls at my school were so fucking horny. Before both my balls had dropped. They were focused. Calculated. I saw one girl at the back of the bus. Pigtails. Hoop earrings. Sat right in the fucking middle. Alpha shit. She asked her friend to call her and then shoved her phone down her knickers.

School French trip. I'm 11. Back of the coach. I'm surrounded by girls. Five or six of them. I'm the only boy pretty much. Played in the football team or whatever.

Truth or dare. Every dare is either to do with a teacher or my penis.

I dare you to call the teacher a cunt or put your hands down his trousers. Or for me it would be punch the coach driver in the nose or suck this Polo from Tayler's cleavage.

I was stunned. Excited. Unsure. I didn't even have pubes then. One of the girls would pull her hand out from my trousers and start describing my penis to the others sat around me. The length and width. I can't remember if they got down to my single ball. I was just supposed to enjoy it though. These were the popular girls. But it took a while for it to click. I hadn't experienced those urges. Wasn't interested. And the girls that age loved it. Couldn't get enough of my lack of interest. But by the time my hormones kicked in and my second ball dropped, they'd moved on.

I got bullied into a relationship once. This girl who had spent the first year of school throwing popcorn at my head. She was part of this girl clique. Fake Burberry crew. Short ties and black pumps. Couldn't believe it. Got a text one day from the leader.

Du fanc Gracey? She wants 2 go out wit u

No. She throws popcorn at my head I h8 her

Go out wit her or well make ur life a living hell

Kk I'll go out with her

I agreed out of pure fear. Spent two weeks ducking through corridors, diving in and out of lessons, doing everything I could to avoid her. I figured if I could just swerve her for long enough, then she'd break up with me and it'd all be over. But one time, after detention, I walked out into the playground. A hundred years between me and the exit. Big parka jacket. Overfull backpack full of shit I didn't need. About to get the bus. Look to the right. Burberry crew. Right there. On the steps by the entrance.

One of them shouts over, 'Hello! Gracey's here! Why don't you come and give her a kiss?'

'Nah, I'm ok, thanks!' I say, pulling up the straps on my bag. Extra speed.

Then she says it. 'What?! Are you frigid?'

The worst thing to be in school at that time. Meant you weren't down for being sexual. A prude. Fuckin' loser. Cut through me like a bike in traffic.

'No . . . I'm not frigid.'

'YOU'RE FRIGID!'

Breathe out. Concede. I bumble over to them. Lugging my bag. Gracey is there with her straightened hair, plucked eyebrows, gluey lips. She's sucking on a drumstick sweet. She sees me and pulls it out of her mouth. Her friends squeal around us. We both lean in for a kiss. A snog. Mouth open. Tongues out. It's fucking awful. Her tongue's like a washing machine. And when we pull away from each other, a long bit of spit runs between us. I say my goodbyes and dart. One of the crew follows me out for a second. A nice one. A girl I'd end up fooling around with but accidentally putting my finger in her arse. She asks me if I enjoyed it. I say, 'Not really,' then get on the bus. Get home. In the bathroom. Wash my mouth out. Soap on my tongue. For real.

In my world girls didn't give a fuck back then. Or they did, depending how you look at it. It was only when we got a little older. Towards the back end of secondary school. When boys' bodies grew. That the dynamic changed. Boys' bodies, maybe not their minds. And the competition was wild. Boys would go round saying that they were 'good in bed'. Like they had a sex algorithm. No way. Pubescent peacocks. Sex collectors. Conquest for the easily persuaded. Were we in control? Did we have power?

All I knew back then was that I knew nothing. Sex education was a load of shit. Some old guy telling us not to wank and then finger a girl straight after. A fucking VHS of *Johnny Condom*. My computer had enough speed to load sexy desktop wallpapers. Glad I didn't learn from porn though. Can't imagine what's going on now. But there was no instruction. Total taboo. Had to learn through trial and error. Hope for the best. Weather the rumours. I had all of them. Every fucking rumour. And they all hurt. Boys and girls. All loved it. Feeding on mishaps. En masse. Vultures in smart black shoes. School policy. Reputation. Hierarchy. Yeah, we learnt about power dynamics in the playground. After school. Punch-ups at One Stop. You get older and the playground gets bigger. But none of us knew. And we came from an age where girls found keys. They knew our secrets.

They could determine reputation. They knew what boys' dicks looked like. They knew what boys were like. What they liked. How they acted. A safe of secrets. And I wonder if that added to the angst. Mutated the fear a bit. Maybe boys were scared. And so tried to control situations in the way they could. Bravado. Belittling. Repeated cycles.

Pressure perpetuated on both sides. Can't cum quickly.
Got to have a big dick. Know what to do. Find the clit.

Boys would spread their wings, flap at each other, scream,
'Come on then!' Butt heads. Girls would join in, egg on,
holler if it got out of hand. Domination. Animal, now I
think of it. A Hadron Collider of invisible laws. Whole
body conditioning. Filling in the blanks. Picking up the
baton. Who's got the power? One thing I will say, you
don't want to be top of the food chain at school. I don't
think so. It warps reality. If you're the big boy bully. Get
your lovers, win the fights. You leave school and find chaos.
Misery. With no backbone. No personality. A big fish from
a small pond that's swum into an ocean.

Sexually I didn't want to dominate. One of my secrets.
I didn't mind it. Had the body for it. But had a crease in
my shirt. A kink in my fake Ralph Lauren. When I was
little. Really little. 6, maybe 7. My mum would go round
to her friend's house who had the same name as her. That
friend had a daughter called Verity. And Verity had a friend
who looked like Björk. Björk was a little older than me,
I think. Definitely taller. One early evening, when the adults
were in the kitchen weighing green flowers, Björk and I
were in the bedroom. Verity wasn't there. We role-played.
She sat me down in front of the tiny little black telly
hooked up to the Super Nintendo. Wicker chair, one foot
tall. Shit posters. She pretended to be an evil queen. Found
a bunch of Verity's bandanas. Started tying them around
my little wrists. Stepping around me like a music video
from the mid-noughties. But it wasn't even the mid-
noughties yet. I was overcome. It felt so fucking good to
be tied up. And terrifying. Which is more exciting. We

could hear someone heading towards the bedroom so she quickly untied my legs. Left my arms tied though. Took me into the clothes cupboard with her. Put one finger on my lip and said, 'Shhhh'. Very Björk. I didn't know what that feeling was then, but I loved it. Utterly powerless.

Having my arms tied became a thing. I asked all my friends at that age to do it, and at that age they were all girls. I used to get erections. Had no idea what they meant but somehow I knew it was forbidden. I knew that we shouldn't let anyone catch us. I don't know why I knew that. Regardless. I wanted the ropes tied tight. Tight enough to squeeze all infantile pressure from my fingers. Tight enough not to feel responsible for my mum's happiness.

*

I'm in Rio reading tweets and tweets. Articles. Statuses. Pictures of statuses. Awful men. Foul, reprehensible men. No knowledge of consent. Pure entitlement. I know, I know, I would think. It's fucked, I would think. I get it. I get the anger. It is fucked. Some of the stories were sickening. Some less so. There were glints of confusion in regard to people's individual responsibilities. A good friend of mine said she felt infantilised by some accounts. As if she, as a woman, had little autonomy. She was proud of her responsibility. Her judgement. And had accepted when it faltered. She's been through a fucking lot too, to be fair. But generally this time felt like an overdue fire. It made sense. And I feel fucking wide open. I have a lot to dwell on. Deal with. Wanting sex more than anything. Betraying partners. Lying. Struggling to commit. Blaming lovers for my own bullshit, I must add. This isn't specifically a 'male' thing, but it's true to me. And I am a man. Just about. Trying to be. Plus with men I find the projection to be more dangerous. The neglecting of issues. The avoidance. And, in all of this, I keep asking myself why this heartbreak is so painful. I keep asking myself why I don't have the tools to deal with it. It's so fucking bizarre to me. How am I in this position? No wonder men kill themselves. This pain's an uncontrollable wave. There's no quick fix. For me, I had no elder reassuring me that it'd settle. And, honestly, if it was just a single elder, I probably wouldn't listen. The pain has multiplied. Two grown men have already suggested I get pissed and fuck around until the pain subsides. Surely that delays the inevitable?

I start to write. I write about how our society informs boys and men on their decisions, or indeed indecisions. Another girlfriend of mine told me that all men have to do is sort out their own community. To accept the fury and step aside. It's worth writing something down. Survival.

26

The Emergency Spiritual Intervention

Gold highlights. Flick of paint. Varnish. Jewellery. Glimmers. My eyes closed. I'm laid sideways on my left shoulder. It's part of the process. Dressed in white. Small white cushion. Flat on the hard floor. Flat white. And I wasn't to move from that position. That was one of the few key instructions. In the white and gold of everything. White food offerings at the foot of the bed. Candles. Calm lighting. It's my spiritual intervention. I'm back in the space. With the sleepy gods. Overnight. Just me in this room, in one position, to be seen to by the energies around me. That's what I was told. I didn't do much, just lay there. Shut my eyes. Couldn't determine what forces were external and what lay dormant in my brain. Couldn't tell the difference between what I wanted to happen and what was happening. Placebo is a powerful force. And I take everything with a grain of salt. So, yes, while I lay with grains of rice at my feet I wondered. And maybe it didn't matter. If I come away from this intervention feeling a bold outer strength, then I win. I never expected to be here. Doing this. I wondered if there was anything else I had to do, but there wasn't. Lie down, eyes closed, let the orishas work their magic. Let the Earth speak to me. I know that my mum would encourage me to keep my heart open. It was the gold that was most prominent in and around the visions I had of prophets and pyramids. Figures I may have sculpted. The gold imprinted. And the next morning, when I was advised not to overthink it. To take it easy. The gold came with me.

I'm reminded by my uncle and the grandmother that what I went through was not a cure. I would not 'feel better'. But it may well have altered the course of my life in the coming months. Basically, regardless of what had happened I will still feel shit for a while, and when I don't, it may or may not be to do with my spiritual intervention. Cynicism in the back of my teeth. Massaging disbelief into my enamel with my tongue. They're all very laid-back in spite of the emergency. Must mean that it worked then. I talk on the phone. Scan for difference. In my choice of words or pattern of heartbeat. Interrogating synchronicity.

'When' is such a lovely word. The implication that it will happen is a handshake. 'If' is endless. Another bottomless void. An endless nothing we all pay to avoid. Unless it's followed by 'then'.

*

I wake up the morning after the intervention. Blessed by the grandmother. I check to see if I can move objects with my mind but I still can't. I'm on the bottom of the bunk bed. Premium prison. Uncle's in the kitchen slicing a mango. Grin like the mango skin. Black coffee on tap. Hot and fierce into a small glass. I've got used to that taste of grit. Coffee, bread and nicotine. My everyday. I've started writing about how I feel. What I'm going through. In the hope that men might relate. I've always written to survive. I write things down so that I can figure them out. I saw a poet say that on stage when I was a bit younger. I'm often not even sure what I've written until it's finished.

It wasn't long ago that I visited a prison. In London. I was volunteering for a rehabilitation charity. They were granted access for workshops. I was brought in to discuss creativity and the power of writing, then end it with some music. Fucking weird place, prisons. Cast-iron gates, towers. People in cages. Men in cages. Supposedly learning lessons. I pulled up to the snaky castle on my bike, hopped off, handed my phone in. Ushered through the big gates by a big burly bloke with keys by his waist. White shirt, black trousers. Looked like a prison guard. Spoke like one. We arrived in a communal hall or chapel and sat around waiting for the inmates to arrive. I wasn't the only facilitator there. We splintered off into different groups. Began talking. One guy in particular told me he wouldn't write down anything. Never will. I tried to reason, told him that he could burn the paper straight away afterwards. That writing wasn't about being 'good' or writing things in a particular way. It was just about writing. The act of it. The movement. The encouragement we can offer to our own psyche. He got a bit frustrated. Said he's never fucking doing it. I think about it sometimes. All those words stuck in his body.

I write about 500 words – 500 words calling for men to take more responsibility for themselves. For us all as a community to focus on supporting each other emotionally. To not perpetuate avoidant behaviour. To not abuse our bodies and each other. I acknowledge the behaviours within myself that have harmed those around me. My complicity in the culture. I talk about our desperate need to process grief. I send it to Gabriella. She writes up stuff for work all the time. She restructures it for me. Order has never been my strong suit. ADHD again. An under-firing of neurons to the executive functioning part of the brain. I leave it for a bit, sit with it. Which is impressive. Gabriella reckons I can publish the writing as an article.

The day passes and I read the article to my uncle. He's sat at his desk underneath an arch in the back section of the living room. This tropical flat sat on the equator. Rough white walls and clay floors. Dusty slabs. Brick sprinkles that move like spirits through the house. Shower in the bath. Plates in the sink. I read him the article and he doesn't move. He looks me in the eyes. Like he's waiting for a gate number at the airport. I have a very low expectation of the reaction.

He says, 'Did you write that?'

I say yes.

'You have to publish that, nephew. Seriously.'

I pause for a moment and then agree.

I have a fearlessness in this moment. I'm not scared about publishing the article. Because nothing can hurt me more than what I'm going through right now. There's a freedom in it. Where I would once fear critique, saying the wrong thing, now I am not bothered. I've done some writing and my uncle says it's good. Nothing to lose at this point.

Chloe has made contact with a friend. A close friend, Jake. She has directly messaged him in response to something he'd posted, Jake tells me. It kills me. Fucking pierces me. I want to know everything. I want screenshots. How long she took to reply. How often she watches his stories.

Everything. Her response is just run-of-the-mill. No mention of me. La-la-la. Here's a message. While I'm dying. I consider with Jake what to do. Maybe he should ask her to talk to me. Cigarette, cigarette. Jake isn't sold. He'll do it but he's not sure what it'll do. It'll show her what side you're on, I say. Utter panic. I search social media. Check the updates. New photos. New comments. New interactions. La-la-la. While I bend. Split. Splinter.

Here are the other thoughts:

I should be over this by now, shouldn't I? This is embarrassing.

Why do you care so much?

Youdon'tevenneedtoworrysomuchbutyouarewhycan't-youstopworrying?

You're never going to do better than her by the way.

This was your one chance for happiness and it's done. There's no way back from this.

Everything will go wrong from here. This pain could last forever.

She doesn't find you attractive any more and never will.

Chances are she barely loved you anyway and this was all she needed.

I've messaged her.

That's what Jake says. I make him repeat to me exactly how he's worded it. I make him. Every word he says, a holographic connection. A few hours later she responds.

What was she doing in those hours? How much fun is she having? Why is she not constantly on her phone? Yeah, basically she's still not ready to talk. Still feels angry. Respects that I'm going through it but it's not her problem. I guess it's not her problem.

*

A newspaper decides to publish my article. They tell me they're going to publish it that Monday morning because that'll get the most traffic. They think it'll have an impact. I ring Gabriella and I tell her. She's over the moon. Turns out she's going through her own shit too. We talk about that for a bit. Which is nice. It's nice to hear someone else's shit and try to help. Another toxic, nightmarish situation. I'm asking a hundred questions. And everything she says I apply to myself. I put a 'my situation'-shaped piece of clear plastic over every statement and measure it. I say that she should come over here. To Brazil. Some fucking company. How wonderful that would be. A fantasy for sure. I can't get everything that I want. I can't get anything that I want.

*

Monday morning comes. Same, same. Pain dreams. Boring now. Hasn't even been that long in real time. A month, maybe. This shit takes years. That's what it says online. Imagine. Imagine if I feel like this for years. Britain hadn't woken up yet. I'd already eaten breakfast, smoked five fags and sat down in the car park. Let out whatever I needed to let out before going upstairs. I take my phone out my pocket. Start scrolling through my messages. Thumb flick then dwelling. Careful consideration of whose day I was going to burden. Then a message comes through about my article. It's been posted. I look on Twitter. Already people are reposting it. Loads of people are. I can't process it. It's like someone's offering me cake on the other side of a window. And I'm trying to bite the glass. More responses. More texts. Fuck, I'm even getting emails from people I've worked with. Professionally. Professional emails saying they'd read the article. I didn't realise so many people read this fucking newspaper. I waited for the dopamine. It didn't come. Only thing that got me buzzing was the idea that Chloe might read it. And take it as proof that I'm a 'changed man'. Surely it's a possibility. A viral article of my accountability has to count for something. Even just an email. That'd give me a hit. I need that hit.

*

Twelve hours later and your article has been shared over 40,000 times. You're inundated with messages. Messages from boys and men you haven't spoken to in years. Boys who are now men. Boys who used to make you feel small. Cornered. They're reaching out now. They know the wound. People you admire. People who stand for things. They're reaching out to you, personally. They say it's brave. They want you to do more. To build. They're handing you bricks. Serious, sturdy bricks. And you're not even taking the piss out of yourself. Or dancing. Or filling silence.

177

You've expressed something and it's being taken seriously. Authors and thinkers think of you as an author and thinker. Does this mean you're special? That sacred ground. Are you special now? You know how it is in society. You know how the hierarchy works. You're currency now.

What was ultimately an attempt to patch a leak has tapped into the current stream. It's resonated with women who've wanted to understand and men who couldn't find the words. *Newsnight* want to book you. Film and television producers have emailed. Festivals want you to speak. You feel the yearning of your adolescence. Nearly every opportunity you'd been trying to mould has spun into your hands playfully after 700 words of agony. Your phone is ringing but you're smoking another cigarette. In your uncle's car park. So that he doesn't have to see you cry.

27

The Mandy Interlude

A few years ago when I loved drugs – peak hedonism – I found myself in a toilet cubicle with a woman I'd never met. I was directed into the cubicle by a close friend, Geri. New Yorker living in London. A friend with frizzy hair, a husky voice and shocking punctuality. She and I would do drugs together a lot. She introduced me to a load of people. I began to suspect she also loved seeing me hook up with friends of hers. Wild as her pupils and fizzy nostrils. It's a members' club we're in. Dark red everywhere. Waitresses only. Glasses with patterns in. Mottled boozy windows.

'Go in there then! There's a line waiting for you!'

Geri pushes me towards the women's toilets and I just go with it. Stroked a velvet curtain on my way. And then when I get into the cubicle, another woman is just standing there. I wondered what this woman's name was.

'Oh, hi, sorry – I didn't know there'd be someone else in here.'

She scanned me. 'Geri said I'd fancy you.' Rolled note in her hands. Minute's silence.

'Well . . . can I have some of this coke or . . .?'

'I'm not gonna get with you or anything.'

'That's ok.'

We take turns to do the dance. Huddle over and snort. Like scientists investigating. Except it's not an eye socket leant on a microscope lens, it's a crumpled queen up the nostril. Shot of light to the brain. Rush of adrenaline. We turn and face each other at the same time. Snog each other's faces off. Like a romcom. But with the lingering aroma of addiction.

'What's your name?'

'Mandy. We're all going back to mine. Wanna come?'

Yes, I do.

*

Later at hers, a group of us are sat in the kitchen. White light. Fridge magnets. Empty cans. A couple of people also live here. One makes jewellery. Drugs are out, music is on. You know the vibe. Giggles and discomfort. Painkillers. Mandy's stood by the kitchen door. Gives me the eye. I'm honestly too high to fully establish whether or not I fancy this woman but her attraction to me is attractive. That is what I'm attracted to at this point. And she is pretty. But she wants to fuck me and that's hot. And rare. Rare for a woman to be so forward. Honestly, women barely ever look at me. Even if they fancy me I won't find out for ages. Or I'll have to assume something from the tiniest movement. Whereas I feel like I'm always looking at women. And often I don't even want to. I have to remind myself to turn my brain off autofocus. It's a curse. To want to look at women. But only men look at me. And usually when men look at you for too long they want to hurt you.

We go upstairs and get into it straight away. High as fuck. Clothes flung everywhere. Like the same romcom. But with the flickering light of self-harm. Big bed. Queen-size maybe. Lamp on in the corner. Underwear off. Condom on. No foreplay. Feels like she wants me inside her as soon as possible. I want to be there. I usually love foreplay but I just have to go for it. Hope I make the right decisions. Hope I last. Hope I fit. This exchange feels quite druggy. It feels like two people who are high having sex. More swing than usual. Touch more performative. The thrusting is audible. Fuck knows if it's enjoyable. A few minutes in, Mandy pulls open a drawer to the side of the bed and pulls out a bag of pills. We're still going, but she pulls out this bag, sticks her hand in and reveals two round pastel-pink pockets of mystery.

'Eat this. It'll make it feel incredible,' she says.

'What is it?' I say.

'Doesn't matter,' she says.

I agree. I eat the pill. Continue pushing. Try to take it all in. Move her leg. Unsure if that feels better. Woozy. Go back to the initial position. Me on top. I close my eyes for second. And wake up the next morning.

*

I wake up the next morning to the sound of voices. I recognise Geri's voice. A couple of others. Mandy's got to be there. I open my eyes. I'm completely naked. Almost falling off the side of the bed.

'There he is!' Geri says.

I haven't got a clue how I got there. I quickly wriggle into my underwear. Smile with my mouth closed. Geri's more than willing. She waits for me to straighten up and join them on the bed. Recounts the story with glee.

'We could all hear you fucking from the kitchen downstairs. We could just hear these . . . dull rhythmic thuds. Was funny. And then they just . . . stopped. We all assumed it was over but then you guys didn't come downstairs. For a long time. One of us decided to take a look and found you both out cold on top of each other.'

I am shocked.

'You were face down with your ass up in the air.'

Mandy looks at me, grinning. 'Must have been the Valium.'

Must have been the Valium. I thought she'd given me ecstasy or something, not a fucking sleeping pill.

*

We had a whirlwind weekend. I didn't leave the house. No one who was there on that night left the house. We ate drugs and watched films. On the Sunday night I lay in bed with Mandy. Just about to nod off when I remembered it was the *Game of Thrones* season five finale. I leapt up, shouted out to the house and we all gathered around the television. Eventually we left. Bubble popped. Reality seeped in like fabric conditioner. Stomachs like washing machines.

A few days later I was out again. At another club. Engaged in some kind of medieval dance with a woman

I'd just kissed. She kept slipping into the crowd like a Slinky. Disappearing. Then whenever I would see her again she'd be staring right at me. Somewhere across the room. I'd blink, or someone would walk across my line of vision, and she was gone. Very bizarre. Never came to anything. But I was horny and high. And guess who'd texted me as I was leaving the club? I found a 'what you up to?' on my phone screen. A square of chocolate under my pillow. A lemon mint with the bill. I left the club and the sky was lightening. A dim screen. I told Mandy I was heading back to mine and that I'd meet her there.

I made it very clear to Mandy that I had to be up reasonably early the next day so it was a spliff and cuddle vibe. Not drink and uppers. I made that clear. Put it in a text. She gets dropped off and comes up to the flat with a big bottle of rum and that bag of pills. I reminded her of what I'd said. Said that this time a Valium would be ideal. But I'm guessing she didn't want me to be unconscious five minutes after her arriving. She seemed pretty wired too. I asked her if she wanted to have sex. She said yes. Fantastic. She gets into bed. We have sex. She pulls out her bag and asks me if I want that sleeping pill. I say yes, great. I accept her offer and swallow the pill.

A few moments later she questions me. 'Is that it?'

Immediately aware of what I've just swallowed. 'Wait, what do you mean?'

'You're just going to fuck me and go to sleep?'

I can already feel my system becoming gradually sedated. It's a fight I wouldn't win. 'Well . . . I'd already said I needed to sleep. You've literally just given me a sleeping pill?! What else am I supposed to do?'

'I can't actually believe that from you.'

'Can we not cuddle? Like I said?'

'No! I don't want to fucking go to sleep yet, you moron!'

I felt completely fucked. Mandy gets up, gets her shit together and fucks off. Can't believe it. I frown confusion as I deflate and try to figure out what signs I missed.

*

Next day I'm in an Uber. Going round a roundabout. Phone rings. Mandy sounds vex. Asks me why I was such a dick last night. I argue my case. Her tone's lowered. Every word another disappointment. I lean in for a while. Gaze over the edge. Dip my face in. Struggle to breathe. Until it hits me. I zoom out. Clock the painting. I've known this woman for five days. How on earth are we speaking to each other like this? Outrageous. I say I'll call her back. I call Geri. I say why the fuck have I got Mandy on my phone talking to me like we're married? Geri laughs. Says we've clashed sooner than she thought but it was always going to happen. Says Mandy is pretty wild. Comes with the territory. What territory? I say. Do you not know who she is? Geri says. I really don't. I don't even know the woman's last name. Fucking hell. Geri tells me her last name and says look her up! So I do. Turns out she's part of a fucking dynasty. Heir to a multi-billion-pound fortune. I did not know who I was fucking with. I'd been spun. Now I'm in mid-air. Asking her to drop me. The storm was fun while it lasted. She's no longer blown away either. I'm another snapped branch. Another broken toy.

But I was currency myself, at that point. Unaware of it

too. How people saw me and how I saw myself were way out of sync. I had little concern for intention. Dying for attention. Flying around, thrilled. Exhilarating but unsustainable. I knew so little of myself. So what did I have to offer when things got serious? I've struggled to push my shoulders back and stand because I've been so reliant on other people's opinions of me.

28

Well Done for Being a Prick

I agree to appear on a television panel to discuss my article. In London. Meaning I'm going to draw a close to the Brazil trip. I'm going to let go of the yoga mat, panic dreams and shadow boy. I'm going to leave my loving uncle with almond eyes and proper encouragement. I'm going to follow the messages and texts of support. The hope I have to prove my capabilities. Of change. People don't believe I can. People don't want me to. I'm going to follow growth. Break cycles. Pedal through perceptions. I have to let go of the late-night calls and açai bowls. Morning runs to the ocean. The conversation I once had with a stray cat. I'm going to follow my fear and head right back into the energy I was avoiding. Back into Chloe's parameter. Her territory. Back into fresh worry that she's around every corner. Excitement that she's around every corner. Sick in my stomach. Little me in my mind. Deep breaths. New path. Another brick. I've got to build on all this. One continent to another. One life to another. Maybe when I'm back she'll care. Maybe she won't. But all this time I dwell on what went before. Wincing at my own actions. In disbelief of my own neglect. My constant neglect. And now I have to talk about it. Because I wrote about it. I've been unfaithful. I've been toxic. There's little worse than not being able to reverse. So I'm getting praised for this article but I feel burdened. Cursed. And my ego is still desperate. Desperate for Chloe to see me. I still want that more than anything.

*

Back in my bedroom. Carpet feels more beige than when I left. Flat's cold. I can still hear whispers on my pillow. Face in my phone screen. Clicking for highs. Scrolling for clarity. I'd posted some more writing online. A poem. And this blogger writes to me. Her name's FEEL. It's important to mention that she's black because it provided an added clarity. One I wasn't used to. She suggests that I'm self-aware. Wonders how. The poem I wrote was about finding my inner child. I reach back, say that I guess I'm doing work on myself. We talk a little more. Back and forth. Word rally. Feminism pops up. Intersectionality. Race comes into the equation. Race. And as we talk it clouds me. The realisation of my proximity. I always knew it, didn't I? I'm always aware of the differences. But I swing between 'fuck everyone' and 'it's fucking fine'. And it's exhausting. But the truth is my dating patterns say a lot. They say a lot about my upbringing. And my choices have led me into shit situations. Where my race becomes a topic of conversation. Or it's forced on me. And I glaze over. Like a doughnut. Smile like a banana. Yeah, a banana.

Eighty per cent of the women I have been in relationships with look the same. I have an aesthetic type. Which is fucking ridiculous. It's fascist, to be honest. I've obscured my vision, limited my availability. I've cut my aerial in half and tried to look for a connection. Look is important. But I do feel as though I have a responsibility to interrogate how I landed on that look in the first place. My type seems to be tall, cat-loving English roses. For a while this included 'Libras'. The star-sign fascination faded. It was real though. If I was sat in a smoking area with a freckled face and pets were even mentioned, I'd know she was a Libra. My friends know my type. They'd say 'that's a bit of you' and 'makes sense' whenever I showed them a woman I was into. I use girl and woman interchangeably because who knows. Over the years I've slept with women who act like girls and vice versa. Just like me – boy/man. Boy hoping to be man. But always white women. And I'm not white. I'm a bit white. It could be a Freudian thing. Maybe I'm trying to shag my mum. I have spent my entire life with my mum. She's a white woman. Maybe it's a safe space.

Or maybe it's because I spent my teenage years outside London. In a city by the sea. I was one of a handful of black people in my school. Not many more in the city. And all around us was white girls. Some white girls who adored blackness. Brownness. Searched for it. Fetishised it. Worked their way through it. I've had ex-girlfriends google 'mixed-race baby'. Proclaim that they'd never gone black before. And the elephant. The elephant is that even those of us with brown skin. The women with brown skin. We'd hate it. Hate ourselves. Fresh from hours of whiteness on screen, in magazines, history classes. Everything other than sports. The girls would straighten their hair, wear wigs, weave. Hide it. Even contact lenses. We all wanted contact lenses. Brown eyes were too much. Too much brown. How heartbreaking that I didn't even want my own eyes. I really bought them. Green contact lenses. But I couldn't keep my eyelids open when I tried to put them in. This idea of beauty. Sewn into my genes. Massaged into my scalp as a means of conditioning. So I would not think that black or brown is beautiful. And perhaps the love or conquest of a white girl or woman would feel like security. Pixie-looking – that's what a friend said my type was. And were these women capable of understanding the isolation? The inward-facing arrows. The difference. The otherness. It's odd. One of the first people to ever call me a nigger was my first seaside friend. It was like he was trying it out. Seeing how I would react. Most racism used to confuse me. Imagine being told to go back to your own country when you've only ever known this country. Proper trippy. And yet it's hard to hold. Open palm to your partner. It's a lifetime feeling. And I chose partners who'd never felt it. It's hard to break ceilings you can't see.

In fact . . .

A couple of months into my relationship with Chloe, three things happened. First, one of her closest friends descended into a vitriolic rant about how I don't experience any kind of oppression whatsoever and almost spat when labelling me a wannabe victim. I actually found the exchange amusing because I couldn't understand what he was so angry about. Was needless, nevertheless. Also, I'd never called myself a victim. He just asked me if I thought that racism obstructed me in any way.

Second, Chloe invited me up to rural Scotland to party with some of her old school friends. Initially I said yes. To be loving. Then I thought about it. Had concerns. I was confident I'd feel pretty isolated in rural Scotland. Even with her. The idea was lovely, but I wouldn't be comfortable. I'd already made the commitment so I guess I should have said it sooner. But what made it worse. So much fuckin worse. Was that four days before we were meant to go, my dad randomly texts me. Says my Caribbean family are meeting up for the first time in years. That weekend. I sent Chloe the message immediately. Made it clear I'd just received it. And she didn't respond. Stayed quiet. For hours. Eventually we saw each other. And she sighed. Said I should go, but it felt like a concession. And now I was unable to feel happy doing that. I said I'd try to do both. I'd fly back on the Sunday after spending one night with her old friends. No way. No way that was happening. But it became the plan. We travelled up. First night we were there, when dancing, an old woman came over to me and asked if she could touch my hair. Before recoiling and saying, 'Oh, I'm not supposed to say that any more.' I shrugged it off. Normal, to be honest. Why wouldn't I feel different? Plus, it was a ceilidh. A traditional Scottish dance party where people lock arms and swing each other about. It's almost impossible to be sad while being swung around. Like frowning while skipping. Unimaginable. So the racism got temporarily transcended. Or stuffed somewhere in my soul. With all the other bitter realities. Ignorance is bliss. Ignorance is me trying to convince Chloe to dance the night away with her own friends. And then of course I missed the flight to see my family. And, yes, I felt awful about it. Heartbroken.

And then the following morning, sat inside this quintessential country house. In rural Scotland. With Chloe's alternatively educated friends. With their ivy-like desires and green tea. I noticed one woman wearing a gold bracelet similar to one I'd been given by my dad. White woman too. I say I've got one similar. Guyanese gold. She says hers is the same. She has a Guyanese boyfriend. My jaw dropped. Of all the places. I'm in end-of-the-garden middle-of-fucking-nowhere Scotland and this woman is having romances with a man from the land of many waters. Just like me.

I say, 'Wow. What are the chances?' I ask if she's ever been and she says that they're planning to go. I ask her where her boyfriend is and she says, 'Oh, he's just doing other stuff this weekend. He doesn't really know anyone.'

He's doing other stuff this weekend. He doesn't really know anyone. He doesn't know anyone so he's just living his own life. Other plans. No hair touching. His roots are nourished. I felt sick when she said that. This woman had just turned a tap on and cleaned away whatever joy was left in the bottom of the sink.

All of this before the countryside. All of this before the wedding.

A spiral if you will.

Maybe I was angry.

And I must hold myself to account then. For my type. And my choices. Do better to balance my fantasies. Eating an apple on the train while reading a book. But if she's pale, her dad might try and fist bump me.

*

FEEL and I have upgraded to phone calls. Too many words for messages. Better to hear a dialling tone than to see it lost on screens. And we speak. About relationships, love, infidelity, gender. And I say that I've never had a black girlfriend. And she's shocked. And I explain it's more to do with environment than anything. Which makes sense. And culturally, when I came back to London, I felt stuck. Suspended with mid-skin. To quote Earl Sweatshirt: 'Too black for the white kids and too white for the blacks.' She asks if I've ever slept with any black women, and I say a few. I say that I'm not even sure if black women find me attractive. She says that's in my head. But it is different. Culturally. There's nuance. Some additional phrases to add to my love language. I recount a couple of times where these black women would argue with me about foreplay. As if it was a concession. Or that they needed a guarantee that there would be pleasure in return. I'd always under-stood foreplay as reciprocal. Didn't know any different. I do remember getting called a 'bocat' in my teens though.

'You're black. You realise that, right?'

When FEEL says that to me I wobble. It's not shocking. I just don't think I've ever heard a black person say it to me. Feels different. Doesn't feel like a bad thing. When people say they 'feel seen', that's what I feel like now. Seen and heard.

'Yeah. I . . . err . . . I guess I do know that. Hits different when you say it though.'

'I think it's actually kinda mad being mixed-race, you know. Because you definitely benefit from being light-skinned but you don't seem to fit in anywhere.'

'I completely agree. I guess white people aren't as threatened 'cause my skin isn't too dark.'

'Definitely.'

'Mad . . . I'm also convinced that black women don't find me attractive. I never get any vibes. I'm a magnet for cat-loving white women.'

'Chances are you're just looking for different signals. Different life experiences. Different ways of expressing attraction.'

'Yeah . . . fuck. What's going on with you then . . . romantically?'

'Oh, umm . . . I've been on and off with a boy who plays video games all day and has zero ambition.'

'Love that.'

'Yeah, it's awful.'

FEEL's a vibe. We agree to meet up in person at some point. She sends me some art she's working on which is fucking cool. She's got creative juice in abundance. There's a little post-phone call warmth before the cold sets in again.

29

Suzy

I treated Suzy like shit. On and off for six years. Young love. From 18. Time went on. She held on. I didn't push her off. And I didn't grow up. I was becoming successful, soaking in power, so I wanted freedom. And she didn't want to disappear. So it was fingertips. Good sex. Highs and lows. I was blurry. Vanishing. Gender tropes ensued. I tried to buy appreciation. I'd give her phones, iPads, pay some of her bills. Most of the time she just wanted a hug. My ear. But I was vibrating. She cleaned my room. Washed my clothes. And I did fucking nothing. Didn't even know how to. Stunted. My mum was always so stressed when doing chores, it never appealed to me. Looked horrendous. And when I did, it wouldn't be good enough. If I cleaned the dishes, they'd be cleaned again anyway. Suzy was self-sufficient, driven and organised, but caramel when it came to me. Infinitely soft. Which I hated. I hated the effect that I had on her. I often wished that she never cared about me. I was scared of being loved that much. Clearly wasn't ready to be. What I could offer was energy. Excitement. Motivation. Support. I was obsessed with what she could do, how talented she was. She's an incredible designer, and I wanted her to know I loved every pattern, every thread. I would encourage her to put on her own shows, invest in materials, studio time, introduce her to anyone who could help. I'd write about it myself, post about it. All of that. But I'm not sure she needed it.

She didn't need the help. She just wanted a pillar. And I was a nightstand. A nightmare. A bad trip she slipped on her tongue too often. That's what I'm telling myself anyway. There's different ways of looking at it. But I would complain. Nag. Permanently unsatisfied. I wouldn't understand compromise. I wanted her to see things only from my side. I'd attempt to guess what she was thinking. I'd assume that I always knew what was on her mind. She asked me once if I thought she'd be more attractive if she lost weight, and I said yes. Never thought that would upset her. I was careless.

Toys out the pram. I wanted to talk about other relationships I was having and she hated it. Didn't want to hear a single thing about me with another woman. This upset me. We argued. I shouted at her. She shouted at me. Stubborn face. I had a panic attack. First one ever. Fucking scary. Wasn't new to her. She helped me through it. We split. Then she had some bad stuff happen in her family, and I did what I could. Helped her with money, offered her my space, paid for stuff, but couldn't give much else other than that. I knew I was horrible. I even said it. But she never left. Toxic energy. I invited her to a house party I had once. Told her I was hooking up with someone else. Ended up hooking up with her and the other woman before kicking her out. She refused to leave. I dragged her. I couldn't believe she wouldn't leave. I felt trapped. I thought my actions would have been repulsive enough. She just held on. One of many regrets.

The icing on the cake was calling it quits across the dinner table. I was leaning back on my chair. Precariously, balancing on one leg. Chewing on the inside of my lip. She was using her thumb to flick her third finger. Frowning. Her mouth also sideways. Toes tapping. Two people hovering in silence. It was ending because we were in different places. Even with the open relationship. We just didn't look at love the same way. I wasn't experiencing jealousy in the same way as the people around me. And I definitely wasn't possessive.

I had concluded that I was polyamorous. Being that I had no concerns about my partner sleeping with other people, I was open to the idea. Got a little kick out of it, if I'm honest. In my head, the ultimate expression of love was found when a partner had choice. To be with someone who could be with whoever they want, and yet they chose you. Shared everything with you. Would go off with others and come back to you. And I always believed that those partnerships would naturally merge. Combine. Stirred, not shaken. All roads would lead to two. Without hazards or roadblocks. Without fear or prevention. If two people were meant to be together, then what would there be to fear? If your partner is better suited to someone else, why would you want to be with them anyway? Didn't make sense to me. So that's what I believed. Polyamory seemed better suited to my values. Traditional relationships and monogamy seemed too centred around toxic behaviours being seen as a proclamation of love. Jealousy meaning someone cared. Possessiveness meaning safety.

I told Suzy that I felt I was polyamorous and she freaked out. Said she could never be like that. Meant that we were essentially over. Seemed angry that I would say it. I wondered why she wasn't more open to it. Pushed her on it. I do that a lot – push ideologies onto people. As if they're my concern. But she resisted, twisted, expanded. Blew up like a puffer fish. And so the end appeared. And when we hashed it out, it became clear that I was no longer able to hold the grief we carried. I'd grown tired of it. I couldn't understand why all my attempts to throw money at situations hadn't sped everything up. I spoke as if her grief was an inconvenience to me. Living from the neck up. As I was.

I'd said all of this. And then met Chloe no more than a month later. And Suzy didn't find out through me. She found out online. Cowardice from me. Classic avoidance. Dirty clothes in the corner. The illusion of clarity. Headphones in, fire alarms too loud. Chloe suggested I tell her.

Which makes it all the more intense that I've just bumped into Suzy. A week after Brazil. A couple of months into the chaos. I've just sat on a panel, with women, off the back of the article that I wrote. We discussed gender. And essentially I was applauded for making it clear that I was a piece of shit. Or that I feel like I am. We decide to head round the corner and find a pub to sit in. We find one. Typical British pub. Honey-tinted overhead lights, more from fatigue than design. Wooden tables. Frothy glasses. Frothy mouths. Airy conversation. The air is inappropriately light. The tension between Suzy and me feels tight. Held on to. My breath shortens as we walk in. I need a piss so I excuse myself. I need a piss and a breathing break. Gather myself. Align my senses. I wipe some piss off the toilet seat and sit down. Stare at some shit stickers. Uninspiring sharpie squiggles. Get my phone out. Do the social media dance with my fingers. Open up my email. Refresh the page. The mail comes in. And then I see her name. Chloe. At the top of the list. In response to one of the five emails I'd sent her. I'd pleaded with her to understand. Seeing her full name still shocks me.

I click on the email and there's no respite. After a few dutiful sentences, Chloe delivers the final blow. Clear as day. Clear as coral in the Indian Ocean. I will never be part of her life again. She has moved on. I should too.

My arse tightens. I'm in shock. So I stand up, as if ordered to do so, and march back into the pub. Foggy feelings in my wake.

There was a time actually, when Suzy and I first got together, when I stabbed myself with a door handle. It punctured my arm and left a hole. Unbelievable. We were running around her house because I had stolen her laptop. There was a picture she didn't want me to see. We were fucking about. And at one point I caught myself on a handle as I ran into a room. It was only minutes later. When she cornered me upstairs. That we saw the blood trickling down my arm. Staining my light blue shirt. I lifted the sleeve up and there it was. A hole in my arm. I couldn't believe I couldn't feel it. Suzy gagged. My response to seeing it was to march out into the night. In the depths of winter. In Britain. Wearing just a shirt. To walk to hospital. Two miles away. That was my logical response to that situation. Suzy tried to convince me otherwise but

I was set on it. Tunnel-visioned. I was going to walk to hospital. A couple of police officers caught me marching and asked where I was going. I exclaimed that I was going to hospital and then showed them my arm. They recoiled and said I should at least get a cab. Asked how it happened. Asked us if we'd had an argument. I realised how the situation looked and assured them that I had in fact run into a door.

*

'Why didn't you understand all of this when we were together?!'

'I know, I know. I don't know what to say . . . I guess I had to feel like I'd been pumped in the chest by a fucking sawn-off shotgun before any of this made sense to me.'

Suzy continues to press me. Highlights my lowlights and I hold my hands up. All my attempts at unconventional anything have gone out the fucking window. I've got it all wrong. I need to be committed and sure and I need to listen and I need to totally abandon my unrealistic expectations of women and what they like and what they can enjoy and what they want from relationships and I need to stop being stubborn too and so pedantic and restless and annoying. Short breath. Rock in my throat. Suzy is just agreeing. Emphasising what a relief it is to hear me say all this. Then I burst into tears. In the middle of this pub. Literally, our table is in the middle of the pub. I'm audibly sobbing.

Suzy suddenly looks embarrassed, aware of where we are. Pupils glancing either side of me.

I frown. 'Are you conscious of me crying?'

'No . . . no, I'm not, just . . .'

'Just what . . .?'

She wants me to keep a lid on it a bit. And I'm reminded of her fallibility. Her hypocrisy. At times. Not to deflect. Or push away. But it's true: we're all fuck-ups in our own way.

'Do you not think it's weird that all your friends call your mate's boyfriend Daddy?' I say.

'Yes, that is weird but also not that deep.'

'Ok.'

Some sort of resistance. Fight back. Yeah, I'm up against it. Just not quite ready for a total pile-on. And still Suzy moved closer. I could feel it. And a part of me yearns for home comforts. A scar in me wants Suzy's too-much love. But I'm in pieces. And what I want I can't have, which is Chloe's attention. That void. That feeling of abandonment. At least I know Suzy doesn't hate me. Which was on the cards after meeting Chloe and then especially after the article. She decided not to speak to me any more and then the nation did. That's pretty fucked, I get that.

30

Amalie

I'm outside Cookies. Some fucking members' club. Central London. Winter evening. Dark on max. Fag lit. Black taxis. People circulating like blood cells. Red ones, mainly. Padded jacket. Pupils shaking. The sound of the road is almost calming. Tyres on tarmac. Like white noise. Smell of damp pavement. Dry nostrils. Brain's been brutal since that last email. Stuck on nightmare mode. My article's had the complete opposite effect. If she's even seen it. Now I want to hurt myself.

There was one time in the gym, with Jake and Tai, when I was backstroking through my days. Gazing into clouds with glee. Life was my lemon cake. And they were having a hard time. And I suggested that they use their mind to get out of the situations they were in. Convince it to think a different way. Two weights in hand, mid-rep, Jake looked at me via the mirror. Said, 'Your brain's not your friend,' and carried on with the rest of his set.

Couldn't believe it back then. I loved my brain. Together we sang in meadows, zip-wired through canyons. Couldn't imagine not enjoying being in my head. It's where I've always lived. I might have been there more than here. I felt a bit sad for Jake in that moment. To be at odds with himself. And now look at me.

Now my tiptoes kiss the pavement's edge and I'm in my head. Fantasising about walking in front of one of these cars. Logic being that she'll have to see me that way. If I hurt myself. If I end up in hospital. She'll come and see me. I need to know that she still cares. That she ever cared. If she didn't care, she'd see me because it wouldn't bother her. Well, then, I wish she didn't care. Just need to see her. That's the logic. Speak to her. Show her my face in person because energy is everything. I keep saying it. Tone gets lost on screens. We can read messages in the worst tone of voice. The worst part of a person. Just to confirm our assumptions. I always hear the sender's voice when I read messages. Chloe's voice is pissed when I read those emails. Cold. Incisive.

Days pass, and it doesn't get any better. I stop going to tube stations. Just in case. All it takes is one overwhelming second. I try to keep myself around people. Keep myself productive. I go to the studio. Write lyrics. Write songs. Distract. I'm still sober though. And I'm so scared about having sex with someone else. In case Chloe hears about it or changes her mind. Or it confirms everything she thinks about me. Friends and family say that I'm giving her too much power. That I'm seeing my own life through her eyes. Even after she sent me that final email. My head goes to these places. Even with all my new insights from conversations I've had recently, my head still goes to these places. And I think about her fucking other guys too. Which is normal, I guess, but not for me. I've prided myself on not being jealous or possessive. But right now I think about it. Her fucking other guys. A specific other guy. Someone I know. Trying it on with someone I know just to get back at me. Laughing at the idea of ever having loved me in the first place.

Maybe I should fuck someone else. Maybe that'll make it better.

*

My neighbour Lucy invites me to the pub with a couple of friends. Been checking in on me. We sit in the garden. Air's always good. Heaters on our backs. Lucy's friend Amalie is here. The Scandinavian one. Blonde, blue eyes. Aryan. Food's decent. Staff are blessed. I asked Lucy about Amalie the other day. She warned me I was heartbroken. Shouldn't make any rash decisions. But I wonder. Also she's far away. Socially. Other than Lucy, I've got no connections to her. No reminders of Chloe. No loyalties or one degrees. Amalie's in a different universe. Eurocentric, West Central London, popping bottles kind of shit. Sparklers and money. Trap music and spliffs. Everything Balenciaga. She's a genuine escape. Because I've seen people talking to Chloe online. Or there being some interaction. Each one another pin prick. Amalie is out of the way, unbiased, and she lives one floor below me in my building. The least I'm going to do is spend time with her. If I get the chance.

Lucy turns to me. 'Ok, what's your favourite animal?! You have to answer quickly.'

'Umm . . . fox.'

'Give me three reasons why – NOW!'

205

'Fuck, err . . . independent, cunning, mysterious.'

'Great. Sam, your turn!'

'Dog. Sorry. Boring.'

'THREE REASONS! COME ON!'

'Oh yeah. Loyal. Cuddly. Cute.'

'Amalie – go!'

'Elephant.'

'Wow, ok – why?!'

'They've got these really big hooves that can just crush you, you know?'

'Ok. Any other reasons?'

'Umm . . . yeah, big hooves. They're big. And I like their flappy ears.'

'Ok, well done, guys. Supposedly you've all just named what you look for in a partner.'

*

Amalie's flat. Couple of days later. She's smoking a spliff and playing Mario Kart. Something sexy about women playing video games. Why? I fantasise about doing kick-ups with a girlfriend too. An underlying lust for masculinity. Societally. She challenges me to a game and I win. It pisses her off. Also hot. When we talk about my heartbreak she is unforgiving. Can't believe why I am so caught up about it. Why I don't take this whole situation as a red flag in itself. She chucks the controller to the side, slides back into the corner of the sofa, lights up her spliff. Baggy jumper. Mood lighting. Everything's beige. Danish energy. Her right leg's dangling off the side of the sofa but her left leg is lifted and leaning on a cushion. Some kind of woman spread. I heard on a podcast that if a woman finds you attractive, then they angle their genitalia towards you. An invite from the elephant lover. I'm hardly a fucking elephant. But I'll find an excuse to edge closer. Never not exciting, lust. It's dangerous. Extreme. Multi-sensory. The room feels like it's at max volume. Full signal. We both edge closer to each other. Pupils dilated at this point. One more nudge. We kiss.

There's chemistry. She's made it clear she didn't want anything casual. In other conversations. Guess we'll see. She knows. I know.

*

'You've got to have a certain level of arrogance to believe that anyone wants to listen to your writing.'

Got an invite to a party. By a woman outside a poetry event. Any distraction. I've taken Jake. Big tree Jake with comfy branches. He's here for support. The woman's in her late thirties. Tattoos. Sharp cheek bones. Thin glasses. Outside the event the male friend she was with looked me dead in the eyes and said, 'Check out her Instagram . . . trust me.'

Turns out she likes doing yoga naked. Men. The house is ridiculous. Big conversion. Great for guests. Just about the right size for a family massacre. The guests all look like art dealers. There are two groups, actually. The 40-year-old art dealers and then a group of 18-year-olds. Huddled outside smoking. Can't figure the link. One of these 18-year-olds. Young man. Is spitting venom. He's going off on one about how he thinks that his poet friend has sold his soul to capitalism. Gold hoop earring. Harrington jacket. Frontman of any indie band in 2006.

Jake and I are more taken aback by how irate the young man is than by what he's saying. I understand the context. Working for love, not money. Avoiding becoming a cog in the consumerist machine. I get it. A trap we're all stuck in. But this guy's saying he can't even talk to his friend any more. Doesn't even want to engage with him.

I push back a little bit. Suggest the idea that people's opinions change and grow. Perhaps their friendship is more important than any career-based decisions he'd made. Values are important but worth discussing. He hits me with: 'Well, actually there's no point if you think about it.'

'Why's there no point?'

'Because life doesn't really mean anything, does it? And we're all essentially illusions.'

I get it. The fury, the anguish. More now than ever, maybe. I understand it as something deeper though. I feel like there's something deeper going on. 'I suppose the point of existence is for you to assign your own meaning to it?'

He's not having any of it. He goes onto set paths. How we're all powerless to our own destiny. How resistance is futile. How we may or may not be defined by our own karma. How money is no reason to sacrifice integrity. I feel obliged to say I've created for money. The system brutalises us, especially those of us at the bottom. And we're given impossible choices. Sold dreams with thorns. Forced to alter our terms to weather the conditions. However, to some extent, we have some responsibility in

creating the reality we live in. Especially our own perception of it. He's still very angry.

'Why are you so angry?'

'I'm not angry. You're the one who's getting angry.'

Am I? I don't feel as though I'm getting angry. I feel
beaten. I can feel a part of him. I totally felt as though I
knew everything not long ago. Like I was above it all. In
some ways I was. I'd totally cut myself off from the neck
down. My fierce logic kept me alive. If I was decapitated
at that point, my body would have flopped, lifeless, onto
the floor and my head would have just kept on talking.
Feeling is what got me in the end. Emotion. I stopped
running from the roots. It fucking hurt.

'You ever been in love?' I ask him.

'Oh, don't tell me you believe in love?! Seriously?'

Yes, seriously.

'Did you know that schizophrenia occurs when your
brain is overloaded with dopamine. A chemical in your
brain that makes you happy can also turn you clinically
insane. What does that mean? There's no such thing as
love, mate. There are just chemicals that happen at certain
points in your life that someone at some point has assigned
a name to. I can't believe that you believe in love.'

'So that's a no, then?'

'IT DOESN'T EXIST!'

Perhaps he's right. Either way there's a control issue
here. I've learnt the hard way that you feel before you
think.

'Do you write poetry?' I ask him.

'Yeah, why?'

'Can I read some?'

He pauses. Wasn't expecting it. Would he be so arrogant as to let someone else read what he has to say? 'Yeah, ok. It's not very good though.'

'I'll decide how I feel about it.'

He passes me his phone. The notepad app brightness comforting the bags under my eyes. He's a good writer in my opinion. Intriguing word choices. Another pain I recognise. He comes over and sits next to me. I guess this is thrilling, knowing someone's actually reading his shit. I pick up on certain themes. Emotions he's maybe masking with metaphors and similes. Security through obscurity.

'You got a good relationship with your parents?' I ask him.

His voice softens. 'Well, no. Not with my dad.'

'Oh.'

Silence.

*

Boys and beauty. Are boys beautiful? Where do we find it? Frogs, snails, puppy-dogs' tails. That's what we're made of. That's how the old nursery rhyme goes. So we have to find that beauty. We long for it. That fear that we ourselves are not beautiful. A loose thread. Cigarette burn in your trouser leg. These mirrors often show us something cold. We can't blush. And we must be monsters to survive, to be honest. So we mould beauty. Search for its support. And how do we know what's beautiful? It's got to be more than a face, surely. And yet I'm lost in one. The beauty has to extend past aesthetics. It has to. But have my standards of beauty wavered because I don't see myself as beautiful? I'm looking for it outside myself. Watches, cars, women. Goals, gear, girls. Because it has to be outside us. Outside me. I don't know. But I'm spun because of how this person looks. And I need to anchor myself. I have to reorientate my axis. I've met beauty before. In a snappy response. A question. Listen, I have to be attracted to what I see. But I've spoken to people before and their faces have changed. Right in front of me. Beauty springing out of their cheeks. Post-laughter. Post-piss-take. I've seen eyes glow in the middle of a story. I've felt a warm tension from simple generosity. And yet we're flipped over. Beaten. By image. Fantasy. And it's always better in the imagination. Always. We have to anchor, look in the mirror, and remember that boys are beautiful. In a genuine, authentic, leaves-on-a-tree kind of way. In a solar system, sunlight-off-glass kind of way. An undeniable reflection of eternity. We must allow ourselves this truth. Because I wonder how many of our decisions stem from these tales. Tales of puppy-dog tails. Hunchbacks. We have beauty. We just have to connect with it.

*

Me and Amalie have sex. Odd feeling. Great in the moment. Fingers crossed she didn't fake it. Good to feel. Sexual excitement is a core emotion after all. Now the door's opened. It's a bold door, having a fling with a neighbour. It's a door with sharp edges and a weighted swing. Still, I have to move on in some way. I have to edge forwards. My mate says Amalie's gorgeous. I'll keep thinking about that. Says she's much better looking than

Chloe. I'll keep thinking about that. Agan, we're not entirely compatible, but who is? She likes spending all her money on designer boots, wants a child and hates feminism. I consider money to be a false prophet, I'm so heartbroken it's almost medical and am now a spokesperson for sensitive men. Mario Kart's fun though. I can't share too much of her weed because I fall asleep too easily. I start drinking again.

*

One night Amalie invites me out for her birthday. Nothing deep. Few friends for dinner and drinks. I turn up, and the table is half black. Mad to me. Considering she's Aryan and Danish. I'm buzzing. My shoulders drop a little. I'm not saying race is everything. It's really not. But the conversation is different, trust me. The feeling of it. Some questions don't need to be asked.

Unspoken bonds, understandings. Solidarity in response to other things being said. Perhaps it's a reflection of my own insecurity. Or like I'm indebted to my black side, having spent my teens in a mostly white area. But my shoulders dropped. That's all it is. And with Chloe. Like I say, her friends are great. Very intelligent. Compelling. Kind. Generous. But all from a particular walk of life. And awful dancers.

When we get back to Amalie's flat after the meal and drinks, I mention it. I say it's so great she's got so many black friends. I say I love that. She frowns. Insulted almost. Then, in her Danish twang, says, 'They're not my black friends, ok? They're just my friends.'

'No, I know that. But they are black. And I'm saying it's a good thing.'

'I don't see colour, ok! They're just people.'

Sure. She's flustered. Forgot people said that. I keep it moving. Reality is, she does see it. From what I've gathered, all her exes are black. I'm not one to speak of course.

31

Feels Different When You Say It Out Loud

I'm draining my friends. I'm a burden, I'm sure of it. We're in the middle of an escape room. Hotel-themed. Jake and Lizzy scanning for clues, grabbing at the walls. I've never been in an escape room before. Apparently I've got to look for numbers but I just gaze at them. My loving friends trying to keep me distracted. Probably got problems of their own. Lizzy's really good at activities. If there's ever a spare hour, she's on it. Booked. Out the door. Phenomenal energy. They're shouting at me to look under a bin. I pick up the bin and there's a red circle beneath it.

'Guys, there's a red circle here!'

'Great!' says Lizzy. She and Jake use the information to keep moving. What an important red circle. Escape rooms are so methodical. Gradual. Progressive. Not wavelike and chaotic. There's a clear end goal. A set amount of time till the door opens. Rational. Precise. Jake likes it too. I feel like he's in his element here. He likes to feel as though he's moving forwards. I think that's important to him.

It's not the first time he's anchored me. I got into some shit in our college days. That's where Jake and I met.

First thing he said to me was, 'Cool shirt.'

I said, 'It's a jacket.'

And we were best mates. Jake was already at that college before I arrived. Everyone knew him. I swear even the teachers fist bumped him. Seventy foot tall with a heart like cane sugar. Has no idea how good-looking he is. People are drawn to him. But for years he'd hide away. Too many people in one space would give him anxiety. I'm not proud of it but I used to trick him. Tell him there was no one where we were meeting when there were. He'd turn up and have to turn it off. Whatever the worry was. Naive of me, and I wouldn't do it now, but maybe it worked? I feel like he loves a group vibe at the moment.

We don't talk every day. Sometimes we can go weeks without talking. But it doesn't matter. When I remember the times I've been up against it. Just to my right is his tache and goatee. We've laughed and cried. All of it. Not been easy for him either. At all. So I've got time for him. The more time goes on, the more time I've got for him.

But, yeah, in college I got in trouble with a group of girls called the 'Topshop Bitches'. Self-titled. No lies. We went to a performing arts school. They were the dancers. Thing is, I got to be a new person. This college was nowhere near my secondary school. Nobody knew who I was. I had an opportunity to start again. Reframe myself. And I was getting female attention. Which I felt I'd lost. Felt like secondary school was a descending slope into misfit isolation. But here was a bright green leaf. These girls were cliquey. And our subsequent encounters deserve their own book. But in short I got set up with this one dancer. A favourite amongst the group, more shy than the others, but beautiful. Tall, Middle Eastern, calm and unimposing. Never missed a beat though. Always listening. I didn't know what to do. Young confusion. All of that. Meanwhile, where I lived, far from college, I'd met another girl who I was into. But I didn't say anything. I didn't report the news. Jake was one of the only people who knew. Jake was also dating one of the dancers. I tried to hide this other relationship, the one outside college. There was an overlap. Was hoping the other one would phase out. Eventually I got exposed. By the girlfriend I had before! Soap opera shit. She had to do double-agent research to find out. Dramatic tension. She was in theatre. That was what she was studying. So I'm sat in auntie's antique shop. Little one just up from Seven Dials in Brighton. Trying to earn money for croissants. All I wanted was croissants. My auntie offered me some part-time work. I was behind the till. I just had to look lovely, smile when people came in, ask if they wanted help. I spent the initial hours emanating warmth, then I saw Jake's number flash up on my phone just as a customer walked in. I was conflicted. Jake knew I was working. Must be urgent. The customer decided to examine the wall facing me. Turned his back. I picked up the phone, put it to my ear.

Jake immediately said, 'They know.'

And we both knew what that meant. If the TSBs aren't on your side, it's game over. Vultures on the top floor of the main building. Ready to feast on scraps. Cold stares at lunch. Sarcastic smirks beneath layers of foundation. I sat up in shock, phone still clamped to my ear. Auntie walks in. Never asked me back. In the weeks that followed, Jake was my only crutch. With one foot in that group himself, he held my corner. Laughed with me. Constantly reminded me that I had it coming. And he always has since. Even if a few weeks go by without contact. Months even. Busy at work or distracted by books. If shit goes down, he's there without fail. My anchor.

We end up getting out of the escape room in time. We take a picture at the end. I am the third wheel. Rusty. Unloved. But appreciative of the distraction. Even if I do wish I could find a code out of how I'm feeling.

*

Suzy's been checking in on me a lot. She's instinctively had to care for so many people in the past. People close to her. Makes sense. Not sure if it's right, but I don't say no. She still feels like home sometimes. Selfish of me, perhaps. But I'm not pushing it. We arranged for her to come over this evening. And now I'm in the kitchen pondering. My silent kitchen. I'm assembling a wall of denial. Bricks of disillusion. What will or won't happen. Friendly. I'm heartbroken and she cares. She knows my heart. Or at least wanted to. Wants to. Mine, a maze. Hers, a lane. A cul-de-sac. She did not share my confusion of partnership. So now I'm gazing at the kettle. The chipped black dining table. Wishing it was Chloe coming over. Feeling like Chloe is watching me. Looking at an open notebook. I've been doing more writing. All the sentences are too long though. I know that, deep down.

The buzzer goes. I see Suzy's face on the screen. Hear her coming up the stairs. Now she's at the door. Same door she stood at after a night out. Fresh lipstick. Buttons undone. Same doorway in which she teased me about my facial hair. Same door frame I dragged her out of. We say hey and she heads in. Then we dance.

Not literally. We dance around the idea. The inevitable. The truth. I make tea. Each sip shared, another step. I talk about Chloe, but we're still circling. Even when my tongue spins. And I speak again of my sins, I feel the circle. Conversation becomes bath water. Plug pulled out. I'm on the verge of tears and she's right there. Pulls back from the squeeze. She's looking down, then she's looking up and the water runs out. We do what we shouldn't. Something twists. Clicks back. Years of memory, but I'm out of sync. My lips have been trained to a different mouth. Different mouths. So much has happened to these lips since we last kissed. I bet she's wondering if I still have a six-pack.

It all starts happening again. We've done this a hundred times. But my mind and heart are totally out of sync. We're doing this in spite of the circumstances. It's messy. Tangled. I don't know if I'm enjoying it. I ask her to stop.

I apologise, say that my head's not screwed on properly. The more the situation develops, the worse it feels. A cursed Polaroid.

The only person I tell is Jake and he gives me that look. That 'you've fucked up' look. I protest to him, saying surely I'm allowed to have sex. And he says that it's not what I did it's who I did it with. And that I shouldn't tell anyone else about it.

I realise that the action itself has jeopardised my chances of getting back with Chloe one day. I bury it.

*

My mum likes Amalie. She tells me in the local pub. Same one I'm always in. Candle on the table between us. Sweet bread and butter. Doesn't help hearing her say that. My mum knows I still haven't let things go. The music they're playing in the pub is from the seventies. A beautiful era. A time when men often sang about heartbreak. They don't any more. And if they do, it's not very popular. I sip my water and say that I like Amalie too. But I'm not sure it can go any further. My mum shows concern. Rips off a piece of sweet soda bread and nibbles at it. She says that my dad left her in the lurch once. Held on to her in between loves. Felt as though he'd drop her for the other one. That woman was Scandinavian too. My mum worries I'll drop Amalie for Chloe if given the choice. I shake my head, even though she's right. My mum says I'm still giving Chloe too much power. I shake my head, even though she's right. I take a bigger sip of water. Take a look around the pub. One of my old coke dealers walks in and nods at me. I'm spending time with my mum 'cause I slipped the other afternoon. I properly tripped over.

I was on the way to make music. To channel myself. Performative though because I knew I couldn't be too down in front of the producer. I pulled up in an Uber. Industrial place. Battered old cars on the kerb. The hum of distant hammers. I sneak between two cars to find the entrance and my mum calls me. I have to ring the producer to tell him I've arrived but I take the call. My mum's checking up on me. Inevitably worried. I complain. As I have been with everyone. Moan. And I cascade. My soreness snowballs. And my mum agrees, pretty much, with every punch and swivel. But I gain too much momentum.

I tell my mum that I've thought about suicide and her voice breaks. The words leave my mouth. They snake into my mum's ear and she wobbles.

Instantly I can hear tears forming as she says, 'Please don't do that. I wouldn't know what to do.'

And then my voice breaks. Because I can't believe I've just said that to my mother. After providing me with so much life. I really heard those words leave my mouth. And I remember that my life isn't my own. Not truly. I can look at it that way, but it's isolating. Some people lose the fight after fighting bravely. I haven't fought hard enough. And I need to be ok with people loving me. There are people who love me.

I'm sorry that I coated
our memories with pain
Just know that I loved you
more than I loved myself
and I loved myself
so little
that it hurt
to be
loved

*

Haven't spoken to my dad much. I speak to him on the phone on the way to a friend's birthday. It doesn't go as deep as with my mum, but I do tell him how I feel. Red light at an intersection in East London. I'm far from my flat. Feeling flat. Hoping the night lifts me. Brightens me.

As normal. It's been months of this. Months. I'm in a cab but I don't care if the driver hears me. Rain spatters on the window. Lightly. Drizzle. I rub my finger up and down on the glass, making a squeaky sound. Driver gives me side-eye. I'm distracted. My dad is coming out with all this advice.

About cheating. What that does to a relationship. What happens if the relationship starts back up. He's been there. Keeps calling me kid, as he does. I like it when he calls me kid. But can't believe I haven't heard any of this shit sooner. Sounds like he's been through this. He's fucked up before. Had it out with a partner before. I get out of the cab, Dad still in my ears. I'm near the party but I walk the other way. Find a cobbled mews. Sit on a damp step for a second. Roll a cigarette. My dad does not seem hopeful about my situation. I tell him I could do things differently. And at some point I do say, I do mention, the fact he's never shared anything like this with me before. And he says it's because I've never asked. Because I've never fucking asked. Imagine if I'd known what he knows, or heard these stories, before diving into a pool of misguidance. Direction handed to me only through films, magazines and anecdotes. Myths. I never had a blueprint. Nowhere near it. He could have told me how he felt. How it feels. Warned me. Prepped me. But it was never shared. It was Ribena and football. It was jumpers for goalposts.

'Listen, kid, I know it's difficult.'

I wish he felt like he could talk to me. But how would he know? His dad died when he was 10.

*

I call my friend Nina in hope of spiritual guidance. Sometimes she can do it on the phone. But this time she offers to meet me at Paddington Station. A happy middle. Wants to help. Giver that she is. Lover that she is. I turn up. Toy with the idea of eating porridge and sit down. My hunger fades. Only occasionally waves these days. When Nina turns up, she's beaming. Unshakeable. Her personality doubles her height. She asks me to sit down and starts pulling at the air around me. Then breathing exercises. Then visualisation. I always forget to put armour on. She also suggests that I put on some running shoes and run. Keep the energy moving. Then get a bunch of Epsom salts and have a bath. Cleanse myself. Ground myself. She says it's no wonder I've been feeling off. I'm barely in my body. I keep disassociating. And it's true. Day to day when I'm going about my business. Writing, making things, trying to date. It's as if I'm haunting myself. Or there's a helium version of me that I can't tie down. Nina has to leave to get to work. She's gone out of her way for this. Appreciative of help with the charity. The high of her guidance wears off. I go home. I run. I come back. I run a bath, put a shit-tonne of these salts in. Then I sit there. No mood lighting, no candles. Bathroom's got the worst lighting in the flat. Or best, depending on what you need. I'm lying there. I start deep breathing with my hand on my belly, just like Nina said. Then I decide I want to see how long I can hold my breath for. I slide beneath the surface. Now all I can hear is my heartbeat thumping in my ears. My heartbeat and nothing else. A slothy heartbeat knocking at the door. Still unsure if anyone's in.

32

The Bridge to Love

I get an email from a woman called Donna Lancaster.* She runs an emotional trauma retreat called The Bridge. She says she read my article in the paper. Wonders if I fancy taking part and writing about the experience. She says that barely any men take part and she'd love to see more come. I say yes immediately. I go online and see that she does other courses too. One of them is a relationship course. I sign up to that too.

*

Starting to feel myself again. Accepting my invitation to The Bridge was a wake-up shot. A slap in the face. In a good way. Self-love, I guess. I could see light. There's some preparation needed. Namely listing losses. And drawing lines to indicate how severe the loss feels. I put Chloe as the greatest loss. In spite of all the death. I had to collect photos, write down thoughts. It's winter, but I've been cycling. Not too cold. Alarm clock breeze. But my brakes are funky and my tyres worn out. Got enough in them to make it to the local

---

* Google her.

bike shop though. Love them in there. One guy makes incredible stickers in his spare time and always offers me free coffee. Another guy riffs funny stories of his son. It's relieving going to get my tyres pumped. Bikes hanging off the walls. Wheels all around my head. Grins behind the counter. They tell me to come back in half an hour so I head down the street for a coffee. Midday in West London but pretty busy because, like I said, no one really works around here. I walk past a café, do a little people watching, but then stop dead. Two feet facing forward. Motionless.

I just saw her.

I just saw Chloe sat in the café, on her phone.

First time in five months. I'm frozen, and then I keep walking. Running it back in my head. Establishing whether or not it was my imagination. But it's not. It was really her. I tell myself that I shouldn't ruin her day. She probably doesn't want to talk to me. Keep it moving – that's what I keep telling myself as I round the corner. But then I change direction. I've got to talk to her. In person. How could I let up this opportunity? Ridiculous. I head back towards the café. Barely remembering to breathe. Heart buzzing. I get to the window and she's gone. Other people sat in there are staring at me staring at the window. I walk in as if I always meant to. Make it look planned. Order a chai latte. Sit on the seats outside. Contemplating. Adrenaline rushing. Cortisol everywhere. Chance missed. I wonder if it was for the best. And then I see her step out of an off-licence a little up the street. Between the café and where I just was. She's rolling a cigarette. She never used to smoke rolled cigarettes. She steps out and heads off in the other direction. I get up and go after her. When I get to a few yards away

I call out her name and she stops, turns around and smiles.

'Oh, hi,' she says, as if it's the most natural thing in the world.

'Hi,' I say.

I can't believe I'm facing her. I can't believe I'm looking her in the eyes after all this fucking time. Five months of imagination. And her face is still. It almost looks as if she's smiling. She doesn't seem angry at all. This monster-sized huge fuck-off pedestal idea of a woman is now just stood in front of me, arm across her stomach to support the other arm smoking. Seemingly open. Ready to talk. Five months of letters. Zero real-life energy. We've been stood here for a minute and she hasn't told me to fuck off. I ask her how she is and she starts filling me in on her time since. Where she's been. Not too much detail. Just enough to let me know she's been getting on with her life. Career's taken steps forward. That kind of thing. Before asking me how I am, she asks me if I've 'seen her again'. It takes a moment to settle. I realise she's referring to what happened. To me cheating. Asking me if I'd seen her again. Fucking insane to me. My mind buffers. Chloe has no idea. She must have invented a version of me in her head. Looks like I've done the same. Can't figure out if it's funny. When responding to the question I almost choke on the 358,000 cigarettes in my lungs. I rub my eye just to make sure that Chloe is really there and not appearing in smoke like she used to.

I try to emphasise how far from 'seeing her again' I've been. How much my views have changed. My approach and attitude towards love and intimacy. All attempts to fight convention put to bed. Guard down. Total surrender. I believe monogamy works now. I could see myself being married. Fuck my cynicism. Anything to not feel like this again. I'm saying all the words and praying for dilated pupils. She's still stood listening. Still smoking. I don't know if she has anywhere to be. And my mouth continues because I have so much I've wanted to tell her in person. Real-life tone. Real-life body language. I don't want to push too much. I ask about the rollies. She says it's a new thing. Rolls another one as a car pulls up for a couple of minutes. Moves on. She tells me a little about her travels. I'm scared to ask if she's seeing anyone. She doesn't mention it. We shove five months into forty-five minutes. She stays longer than I expected. No further plans are made. Another car pulls up. She says, 'This is me,' and gets in. Then it's, 'See you around.' And the car pulls away.

An anchor descends from the sky. Travels through my skull. I go and get my bike. Pedal back in shock. Realise I forgot the chai latte. When I get home I burst into tears. Proper gut tears, this one. Gutter tears. Belly fucking ab workout. I'm reminded of the base-level dislike I have for myself. That beneath it all. Beneath all the comedy and performance and charm and wit, I hate myself. I sit in tears and repeat it to myself just as my mum had done. During her panic attacks. Just before the paper bags became a parachute. The ones I'd save from the shop.

*

It's a couple of days later and I've left the gym. I've got a few things to sort before I set off for The Bridge on the weekend. Phones are locked away the entire time. Which

I'm looking forward to. But it takes a little mental prep. The pain of Chloe coming and going still rings in my ears. But I know I need to reset my focus. And that The Bridge will be a golden opportunity to let go of this shit once and for all. I'm briefly overcome with a sense of freedom.

Then my pocket vibrates.

I take my phone out of my pocket and see Chloe's name on the screen. Again, doesn't feel real. I have not seen it in so long. Too long. I gather myself and open the message. She says that she knows I'm about to go away but maybe we could grab dinner before.

I feel sick.

*

The retreat was in the middle of nowhere. Just like me. A beautiful, detached farmhouse. Dirt roads, no signal, pigs out front. The scent of fresh manure still feels cleaner than city air. Would rather breathe in cow shit than car fumes. Couple of cars pulled up already. Welcomed in. Feels like the first day of school. Big green trees surround us. Standing people. No phones for the whole six days. We can smoke but it's not encouraged. The intention of the week is to remove all barriers between ourselves and how we feel. I'm one of two men in a group of fourteen. We're all about to surf together. All week. First night, I'm already doubting. Fucking hell. When we share our losses and I hear some of these stories, I start to think I've got this wrong. I shouldn't be here. My grief's a bit pathetic in comparison. Some of the shit these people have been through, and I'm here upset about my gran dying and a fucking breakup. I voice my concern. And one of the facilitators, one of the angels, says that grief is incomparable. That I should continue on through the week. And to trust her. Which I did. I saw the thousands of people in her eyes. Spectrums of pain and healing.

The idea is to travel into ourselves. Every day we are to move. Shake our bodies like dogs. Reset. And some were very conscious of the group dynamic. Aware of others. Total strangers. Showing our largest wounds. It's unusual. But as the days progress, the connections begin to deepen. We begin to merge into a single organism. Not without resistance. The yawns get bigger. We start getting headaches. Migraines. All types of stuff. Our bodies are cleansing. Pushing shit out. Flaring up. I had no idea that emotion was stored physically until I did this. It's literally stored in my body. A back-up of grief. No wonder people get bad backs. Dodgy knees. Especially men. Secrets in our shoulder blades.

Being that we don't have our phones, I dream without distraction or relief. No immediate comparison. No fear of missing out. No nothing. Just heartache and white blood cells. A cold pillow and razor-sharp dreams. Uncut DMT. Every night. It's hard to sleep sometimes. I'm sharing a room with the other man. He lies there with regret. That's what's keeping him company. Every day we're encouraged to walk out into nature on our own. Community and solitude are to be in balance.

So I walk out into the long grass. Think of rap lyrics in between daydreams. Or as an escape. From what I'm too scared of confronting. I escape into rhyme schemes and word patterns. Like I always have. Run my hands through straw. Less effort with every returning journey. And I continue to build. We continue to build. We're building towards writing two letters each. To whoever we feel we need to. Dead or alive. Letters that are designed to release the tension. Charm the trauma out of you.

We're asked not to comfort anyone during the six days. Caretaking, they called it. No caretaking. Really fucking hard not to do that. We're all on this bridge journey, watching each other cry every single day. But no touching. No hand on the shoulder. Nothing. That kind of reaction is impulsive. Certainly for me. Second nature. I want people to feel better. I want to be the reason people feel better. So they'll like me. So that I can feel like a good person. And because I care.

We're split into two groups. Each run by one of these experienced, gifted and enlightened women. Powerful fucking leaders intent on metamorphosis. Having been through their own shit. And now we're wading through our own shit.

I pull my leader to the side and say, 'I'm unsure about these letters. I thought I was going to come here and move past my biggest loss, which I've put down as my ex-girlfriend. But I saw her last week. For the first time in months.'

'Well, I'm happy for you! And don't worry about it. Believe me.' She smiles at me. She's seen a thousand bridges. And here's me distracted by a little piece of string. Like a cat.

We're learning to love ourselves. An impossible task, surely. To truly value the self. So much of society encourages us not to. It's suggested that we learn a lot about ourselves in relationships. Intimate relationships.

Some stuff that stayed with me:

- Relationships generally work in stages. There's the honeymoon phase, then there's the power struggle. If you make it through that, there's growth, and way down the line there's a thing called 'passionate friendship'. According to some studies, staying with a partner for a long time results in our brains emitting a constant supply of oxytocin. Which might explain why older people 'die of heartbreak' when their partner passes on. Over 60 per cent of relationships end after three months. When the high of lust fades and the reality of the power struggle kicks in.
- Partners should only be responsible for 25 per cent of their partner's emotional struggles. The majority of the initial responsibility is up to the individual. We must take control of our own lives.
- Shaking genuinely helps relieve the body of anxiety. All animals do it naturally. Stretching too. An everyday necessity, no question.
- Learning to identify where we feel emotion in the body can help us move it along.
- In relationships there's usually a 'maximiser' and a 'minimiser'. A maximiser very much wants to deal with issues head-on and in the moment. A minimiser prefers some time to reflect. Arguments are rarely solved unless there's acknowledgement of the difference. We often end up seeing our partners as our parents. Even if we don't want to. This is called a 'transference trance'. And it's our responsibility to be aware of it.
- Most relationships are destined to end once critique, passive-aggressiveness and judgement slip in.

- It's imperative that we say no when we want to.
- Sometimes we're acting from a place of unconscious loyalty to our parents. For example, a person might jeopardise a relationship whenever it gets serious in fear of losing a connection with their mother.

We're all building up to these letters. I write the first one to my mum. I read the letter out and I have a trauma response. Sobbing. Can't stand up. There's a way to write these letters that helps summon trauma. Like a rattlesnake. Helps a person stop feeling like a basket case. Scaffolding. Or some kind of lift. Cleaning a window. There's a structure to it. And the goal is to write without thinking. We read these letters out to facilitators who are responding as if they are them. Whoever the letter's written to. Easier to imagine than you might imagine. And the trauma rises. Like heat. Tears out of nowhere. Turns out most of my trauma was hiding in my right knee. Pain trapped under my patella.

I realised while writing this first letter what my main grief was. It was just a sentence. A throwaway sentence in my mind. The sentence I thought about the least. But in that moment, I'd tapped in.

When writing, physically, pen to paper, I'd hit the well. It was because of the scaffolding. Next day, we're asked to start preparing the second one. I shuffle around the main room tapping my lip with my pen. Pondering. Humming. Gazing at the trees through the back doors. Green through glass. Dreaming. One of the facilitators walks by and asks me if I'd settled on my second letter.

'I'm not sure . . .' I say.

'It's a tough one,' I say.

She nods. Gives it a second. 'I think you should write a letter to your dad.'

Then she leaves the room. And I'm left. With a noise. A muted tone. The kind of sound you play to make youths disperse from an area. A sound to make you change channel. Something's wrong. No words. A blank expression. Face scrubbed. A sparkling silence.

I write the letter. Read it out. Burn it. After I read it out loud, I have another trauma response. From a sentence formed when my mind wasn't in the way. When I let my body do the talking.

Different though, this response. Trauma gets thrown around these days. The word itself too. This is a different branch of it. It's primal. I can't speak until I scream. Roar. I have to be restrained. Held. Told to let it out. The energy's different. I'm angry. Full of rage. Having a tantrum. Blurring the line between child and adult. That's a lot of the work, actually. Listening to your inner child. They never lie.

Your
body
knows
the
time
Matter
over
mind

We burn these letters. And create altars. Confront symbols and memories of our past head-on. We open ourselves up to being loved. Maybe the hardest part. I hate it. Being sat in a chair receiving compliments. So difficult to accept love. With every message from the group a voice in my head would tell me it's bollocks. A violent voice I've picked up along the way. Not my voice. But I push through it. And it means the world. My world was changed. Most of my Earth time has been spent trying to show people I'm lovable. Then having no clue what to do if they believe me.

I feel physically lighter after the six days. I've confronted a couple of wolves for sure. Namely my parents. Specifically the complex, intergenerational layers of emotional debt. The cutting of ties. Unconscious loyalties. An awareness of where my actions are coming from. And why they're happening. My patterns of self-destruction are of no benefit to myself or anyone around me. I actually want to change that. I want to connect to authentic anger. That healthy, core feeling. And feel better for it. I want to give myself some love in this moment. Hug myself. I have to acknowledge that for all my fuck shit. My failed intimate relationships, attachment to perpetual sexual validation, drug abuse, failure to commit, impatience and avoidance of stillness. I want to look ahead, talk openly with my parents, look after my body and breathe. I've turned up to this retreat wanting to change. And now my future feels hopeful. Every morning now I want to move my body. I'm high. A really fucking natural high. I've abused my dopamine receptors for so long I'd almost forgotten what this feels like. I'm climbing a ladder at full speed. Infinite up. A clean high. Body high. No chemicals. I've been kicked out the nest but I've flown. I'm a rat with wings.

I'm lighter and brighter. Six days done. My new family

are now leaving. Vulnerability breeds connection. I know that for a fact now. I feel a deep bond with this group. Would go out of my way for them, having only known them six days. How does that make sense? But if I deep it, many of our strongest bonds are birthed in these moments. Whoever's there at your 'lowest'. You never forget that. I get my phone back. Turn it on. And the first thing I do is message, Chloe. The minute I get an opportunity. The first thing I do, with this newfound bounce, is run to her. I thought about her a lot. Every time I had a breakthrough. I'm wondering if it'll change things for our future. I wonder if she'll be able to feel my change of energy. I'm in wonderland. And even with the tools to climb my way out of this, I can't help but bounce back into my rabbit hole.

32A

Smoky Father

Like I said, I burned the letter to my dad. And that was important. But if I was to write another one, it'd go something like this.

Dear Dad,

If I could drink the silence between you and I, it would taste fizzy when it shouldn't. A fruit squeezed pure. Carbonated through avoidance. Bubbling on a dry parched tongue. Desperate for conversation. Condemnation. Boundaries, life lessons, limes, lemons, fucking vanilla ice cream. A palate cleanser. This shit's too bitter. I want to share some air with you. Climb a mountain. Shiver together. I want you to remember me whenever you toke on your cigarette. And the cherry glows. Evidence that breath can bring light to a situation.

We've spoken more recently. I came to you. I had to. Silence is a spectrum. The dial was way off. And I miss you. Every day. I want you. I love everything about you and respect what you've been through. I'm angry about times when I haven't felt more important than everything. The little me doesn't care what you went through. What you've survived to be here. Little me just wants affection all the time. And compliments. And ideas. Of course, I got them from you. I remember every gift. Vividly. More than I can remember myself. I'd see you but know nothing about you. I'd guess. Pick up puzzle pieces from my mum. This big great mystery who I adore. Stories intertwined amidst your big dreadlocks. Desperate to understand my roots. Even if there are twisted truths.

I remember those Ribena juice drinks so well. My mum didn't want me to have those sweeteners in my stomach. Said they were toxic. But every child wanted it. A dopamine injection comparable to cocaine. You would hand me this addiction as if to say 'I love you'. As if to say 'My love for you is more important than your health' or maybe it was more 'Please love me. I'm unsure of what love is'.

So I would finish these drinks as a way of saying 'I love you' back. Sometimes instead of just saying 'I love you'.

Then I'd go home and throw up

Everyone blames their parents for everything. Everything is everyone else's fault. Maybe there's no blame. Just a need to vent. No one's perfect. And we're all drowning. In survival mode. Some of us never got to grow up. How do kids raise kids?

When we sat, that night. Winter. Cold ashtray. Lights kind of dim. You said you felt as though I had been passive-aggressive with you. That for years I'd said and done things in a particular way. Slight you. Undermine you. Sometimes in public. Very rude. And I said, 'Yeah, I fucking did. I fucking was passive-aggressive. That was the best I could do. To deal with anger.'

You felt that.

I said, 'I actually don't give a fuck how I've been with you 'cause you're my dad. You can tell me I'm out of order. Discipline me. But say it then. Don't be upset by it. I want you to be a big building. I don't know if that's unfair. I want to throw rocks at a big building. A big building that gives great hugs. Do you know what I fucking mean?'

You totally got it. And then we connected. Again. It must be frustrating. To have a son who questions everything. But you have one of my favourite smiles. I feel full when I see it. Lights up a room. Your laugh too. And you're so talented. I can't believe you never taught me how to play guitar. Actually that's bordering on unforgivable. And you're wise. And sensitive. So why have I got to drag it out of you? I want all the knowledge. And all the joy. I hate the way you eat though.

From J

33

That Boy Shit

Talk men, talk silence. That quiet pain. That forever pain. Stored inside. Cupboards full of curses. Kept shut under the guise of courage. We're taught to fix, not surf. Saying that, we'd take laughter over silence any day. But our laughter is a special kind of silence. We avoid discomfort. Stillness.

Sometimes I wonder if we feel more. As men. Which is why we go to such lengths to disconnect from it. Because it's too painful. And we have to fight. On top of that. It's a cruel system. Can't appear weak. So often the truth is muted. Kicked under the bed. Forced down to the bottom of the bag. Even if, in truth, expressing pain is truly fearless. Even if surrendering to pain is the only route to maturation. We've decided to hide the conversation. Code it. We get it in the ear about our chosen languages but they're pure. There's some beauty in them. If only they lived alongside a freedom to express and explore. Without fear. One language that a large majority of us speak is football.

Men. Football. Hooligans. Racism. Yobs, yeah? Hardly adverts. Football is a working-class sport. Kick a ball and you're in. Once you're born, you have a team. A lack of money's less painful when you've got passion. No club membership with football. There's barely any equipment. Jumpers for goalposts. No 'etiquette'. When you've been kicked around, what do people expect in return? Is there any better theatre than football? No suits, just home shirts. Half-time interval. And anyone can go for it. Anyone can climb the ranks. Blessing and a curse. A curse for the 93 per cent that don't make it. But if you do. Theatre of dreams. Your name being sung by thousands. You've got to be in a stadium to feel it. And suddenly all this love comes gushing out of the silence. All this noise. A ball flies into the net and people fly into each other's arms. Strangers hugging strangers. Collective grief when the team loses. So much of our souls lie with a badge. And what for? It's just that boy shit. A rush of blood to the head. Winding each other up. Got to watch it doesn't fuck your life up. But every now and again, there's an unmatched sensation.

In 2012, I went to see the Arsenal FA Cup third-round match against Leeds. We were at home. I'm an Arsenal fan. Long-suffering. Not for much longer. The game was fairly innocuous other than one important detail. Thierry Henry. Arsenal's greatest ever player. Had returned to the club. Past his prime at that point, but he could still play. A god amongst men. I'd imagine that I was related to him sometimes. Tried to buy the same boots as him. Mimic his celebrations. He played with flair and confidence. A shooting star. Literally. After his original, unforgettable years at Arsenal, he left to play in Spain. Now he's back. He was so good at football that even fans of rival teams loved him. A magician in knee-high socks. In the seventy-seventh minute of the game, he's brought on as a sub. It's nil–nil. Arsenal on top but not finishing. Henry's on for about four minutes before he makes a run behind the defence. Not just any run. His kind of run. He even had his own run. The ball is played in perfectly by a player called Alex Song. Song by name and nature. Henry opens his body up so he can strike it with his right foot. He does. And he scores.

Honestly, the energy. If I could bottle that up, it'd be banned. It'd be classified as Class A immediately. Even the Leeds fans were singing. Sixty thousand people were cheering and singing, 'Thierry Henry, Thierry Henry!'

All that joy circulated the stadium. It left mouths and entered hearts. Strangers were hugged. All that energy vibrating in the air like bouncy balls in a washing machine. All different colours. I can confidently say it was one of the best moments of my whole life.

And imagine the reach. The reach of these teams. The extent of passion. Our society suffers from a severe lack of ritual. Where else can you hug like that? Embrace. Football is far from a male-only sport. Biggest Arsenal fan I knew growing up was my mum. Nowadays it's my friend Dee. She fucking loves it. But it's a worry how long men can go without intimacy. Some kind of feeling. Being held. Rejoicing. We need feeling to be alive. Babies can't develop without it.

There is such a backlog of energy, it can flip the other way entirely. Manifest the worst in us. A bad result can ruin entire days. Entire relationships. We struggle to moderate that energy. Because that badge feels part of us. I've been racially abused on the way to a match. I've seen fights break out. People throwing shit, shouting obscene fucking things. Because every high comes with a low. So, yeah, we could do with some moderation. And a filtering out of the emotionally incompetent. I vow to not allow a single thing to rule my life. To solely dictate my emotional state. Perhaps a community a little more in touch wouldn't have to channel so much venom. Because all the words and fury are reflective of deeper issues.

Every day I'm collecting tools to help me channel anger in a healthier way. We've all got to do that. Because anger is important. But left too long it becomes something else.

Still, I can go into a room full of strangers, a shit wedding or an awkward birthday, and all I have to say is: 'Who do you support?'

And we're away.

In a queue. At a club. First holiday with your partner's new family.

'Who do you support?'

On a plane. On a train. In the back of a cab.

'Who do you support?'

And we're off. Horses. A little connection. A spark. The reach of a hand.

Imagine the reach. True story. I once drove through the Amazon rainforest when visiting Guyana. My ancestral homeland, if you can call it that. Moved there from the Motherland. A home nonetheless. There are checkpoints along the way. We pull up. Pickup truck half mud. European anxiety. The checkpoint office is one side of the road, there's a bar on the other. A clearing amidst dense forest. Endless canopy. They've got to check how far into infinity we plan on going. And from what somewhere did we emerge. We walk towards the office and the vibe is tense.

No one says hello. Just staring. Door open, same thing. Three more men. Three more stares. We're trying to offer up these papers as quickly as possible. The fear is that nerves make us look suspicious. And that fear makes us nervous. The man to the right of me is particularly intense. In his uniform. Triple beige. Hint of green. Gun in holster. I figure I've got to do something to break the tension. Take a risk. I clear my throat a little and say . . .

'Arsenal?'

Half a second later, he's alive. The book's open. His eyes and smile double.

'You support Arsenal?!' he says, then bursts out laughing.

'Oh my God, no way!' he continues before jumping up and walking outside. He starts shouting at the handful of men sat in the bar opposite. 'Ay, listen! This man support Arsenal! He's cursed! No way would we support Arsenal!'

Some of the men join in. 'Nah, none of us support Arsenal round here! I support Chelsea!'

Once the officer comes back inside, the energy is changed. Upbeat. Kind. Like we'd unlocked a new level. Just by whispering a football team. In the middle of the Amazon jungle.

*

Then there's the attempt football makes between father and son. To create some kind of conversation. In an ideal world, this runs alongside authentic connection. Alongside honesty, clarity and support. We might not be there yet but we're trying. There can be translation.

It's a Sunday afternoon. Overcast. Flashes of sunshine.

Father arrives to see son. Hasn't seen child in a while. Busy with work. A little bit scared. Father's feeling things he doesn't want to feel. Doesn't want to burden the child. Doesn't want to feel burdened by the child either. Tricky game. Child's happy to see father. Overjoyed. So plays it cool. Pretends not to be that bothered. Quick hug, maybe. Should be longer. Game's on. In the living room. It's about to start. Five minutes till kick-off. Cup of tea? Cheeky beer? Then the riddles ensue.

Father: How you been then? Alright?

Son: Not too bad, Dad. Good. How about you?

Father: Yeah, yeah. Not too bad. Not too bad.

Silence. Then . . .

Father: So what do you reckon then? *Seriously, how you feeling?*

Son: About what? *Just ask me how I'm feeling again.*

Father: The game. Do you reckon we're gonna win or what? *I know it's been a while but I do care. I've built seeing you up in my head too much. Bit scared, to be honest.*

Son: I mean, fuck knows. We've been shit recently. Been doing my head in. *I've really missed you but I don't want to have to carry this conversation.*

Father: Ha! Tell me about it. But you never know, I guess. That's the beauty of football. It's all part of it. *I am prepared to carry this conversation. And take some responsibility.*

Son: Did you see Ødegaard's miss the other day?! Couldn't believe it. *You've got to be better.*

Father: Yeah, that was shocking. I wouldn't play him so deep though. He's out of position. *Ok, this is us hugging.*

Son: Yeah, I'd stick him centre attacking 100 per cent. And keep him there. Did you see when Saka cut in a few games ago and pinged it top corner? *Yeah, let's get into it!*

They both beam a bit.

Father: I'm telling you there's not a brighter talent on the planet than that boy! *Love you.*

Son: He's an absolute baller. You can tell he's sound as well. Runs weirdly though. *Love you too.*

Father: Yeah, he does run weirdly! *Maybe we actually could talk?*

Son: Hope he gets one today! *Yeah, maybe!*

Father: Yeah, me too. He deserves it! *Ok, let me try again.*

Ref's whistle cuts through. Beginning of the game. End of progress. Another hug if they score. Joint groans if they don't. Hope for headway at half time but unlikely.

But it's something. It's better than silence.

I'm so thankful to Arsenal Football Club. For keeping my dad close. Providing neutral ground. A happy middle. For making us present. Locking down locations. Leaving footprints after the final whistle. Footprints we might follow.

*

The other side of the coin is violence. More boy shit. More human shit. We're all violent. Men the most physically violent. Emphasis on physical. Human beings and violence seem inseparable. All kinds of it. Probably because we're animals. And will always be animals. As intelligent as we believe we are, we are part of an ecosystem. We are no more important or superior than a dandelion or a blue-bottle. I don't believe we will end violence. The universe is violent. The ocean is violent. Giraffes are violent. Praying mantises are violent. Venus fly traps are violent. It is nature. I don't believe the issue is violence. I believe that it's the values around it. Honour, duty, sensibility. Mammals wrestle for fun. We just struggle to tame ourselves. Tap out. Call it a day. Too often I hear people claim to be 'pacifists'. As we sit and reap the benefits of millennia-worth of bloodshed. As human exploitation drips from our ceiling. We have the audacity to claim we are peaceful.

I had a mate who used to fight every night we went out. From my late teens to early twenties. I bet you can guess what he was missing at the time, what he wanted more than anything. Love. Connection. Just so happened the next best connection he could find was with his fist. Some drunk jaw. A lazy eyelid. Maybe the restraint felt like a hug. He was being held, after all, in those moments. Even if he was swearing and spitting at people. Still contact. Aimless fighting is a language of the unloved, in my opinion. Or at the very least it's pre-pain. Pre-maturation. Grown men don't fight for no reason. Grown men don't pick on somebody weaker than them or more vulnerable. There's no honour in that.

And I wonder what else lies beneath the chaos. I wonder about the power of words. I've noticed, growing up, that men like to tell other men to 'suck my dick'. They shout it at each other. The same men who will go out of their way to say phrases like 'no homo'. If they fear something they've said might be misconstrued as homosexual, they stand there, arms spread.

'SUCK MY DICK!'

The idea is that it's demeaning. To suck dick. That it's submissive and feminine. But if I'm honest, sometimes I wonder if that's all that these men want. To suck each other's dicks. If I'm ever caught shouting 'SUCK MY DICK' at someone, better know that I mean it.

Violence can be concentrated. Focused. One of the greatest aspects of combat training and martial arts is the discipline. And one of my favourite things that anyone has ever said to me is that 'discipline is rooted in self-love'.

And may I add, while discussing roots, that both silence and violence are found holding hands. In the history of too many. I like to have a rough idea of what's going on. So I read reports and statistics about violence and abuse. I see why there's so much reason to worry. And I also see the flaw in statistics – the ones based on human participation. Who are you asking? Where do they live? There are incontrovertible statistics to highlight the reality of how dangerous life is for women and girls, at home or otherwise. And these findings must have been based on crime reports. Which reminds me that, in my lived experience, if a man has been abused or is stuck in an abusive situation, I'm not sure anyone would find out. The chances that they would report it are incredibly slim. Because the circumstances are different. There's not the immediate threat of death. But there is threat. And arguably little support. I know men who've been attacked with knives, punched square in the face, belittled and tormented. Not all violence is physical, after all. I wonder if gender is reductive when investigating certain widespread issues. Even if there are slants and trends, aren't there human changes that we can all make? As men we need to show up for men more. I'm certain of that. But I also want men to show up for women and vice versa. There are connections deeper than gender. And again, within my pool, it pains me to say it but over half of my immediate male friends have been sexually abused as children. By men and women. I don't know how that measures in regard to wider society, but it's real and it's fucking awful. A lot of what I've read doesn't reflect that. And it's horrendous. And it's taken over a decade for some of these truths to come out. Burying trauma like that is a life sentence of its own.

*

But let me not add to the noise. Because men are talking more. Chatting. Podcasting.* Enquiring. And the noise created in the corner overshadows the room. We have an abundance of great fathers, partners and mentors who work with a different silence. Under-appreciation. Songs unsung. The nuclear few attract too much attention while boys don't grow up quick enough. And so the saga continues. I wonder if we pay enough attention to the beauty. The masculine beauty. The immovable core. Duty, honour, respect. Those aren't lost promises. They're ancient compasses. North Stars for the soul. There's a man who lives down the road from me. Forget his name. Middle-aged. Happy cheeks. Curious wrinkles. He's got a little black shaggy dog, and every Sunday he goes along to our local park with a litter picker and picks up all the rubbish.

* Questionable.

Then comes home to his partner and children. No fanfare. Just honour. He puts on a balaclava. Sabotages fox hunts. Comes home. Makes dinner.

And the term 'masculinity'. A firm indicator of that boy shit. Flows beyond us and our bodies. Let us remember it's an energy that can become toxic and extreme like all energy. Anything is damaging if taken to an extreme. Anything. Even broccoli. Look it up. Femininity. Every energy exists on a spectrum. With sliding scales and a pull towards balance. Our current society is so biased towards traditional masculine ideas. Which is to say. Invented ideas and what it means to be 'a man'. That perhaps we lose track of the responsibility we have to nurture both energies within our soul. Remember that a human can channel both. At any time. We can uphold ideas that damage us. I've searched for peace with my femininity. Actively engaged with it. I grew up around women. But too much so. I've craved my masculine energy. Needed the other leg. I'm no flamingo. And imagine my confusion as a young boy seeing my mother screaming at the television if Arsenal were losing. Driving faster and more dangerously than anyone I know. But never crashing. Parallel parking with ease. Smoking twenty Silk Cut while fighting the powers that be.

First time a girlfriend sighed when the football came on, I couldn't believe it.

34

A Year After What Happened: Part Two

Chloe is my girlfriend again. Yeah. Unbelievably. After The Bridge we started hanging out again. And I was hanging on. Felt indebted. Couldn't believe it, that I had another opportunity. Jake was in shock. We all were.

Started with a dinner. Proper nervous. Didn't want to put a foot wrong. We took it slowly. Which meant we skated cautiously into Valentine's Day. Valentine's Day arrived right at the point where we had had a few more dates. Felt ourselves twist into each other. Played cards at the pub with no expectations. So I had to pull out the stops. My chance to impress. I turned up to meet her outside therapy with a confetti cannon full of hearts. Bought us cat onesies. Played around a bit. Went to a gig. One of our favourite artists. Moved towards touching for the first time in months. I was really trying to gauge what was appropriate. But the electricity was undeniable. Taboo too. Shouldn't be happening. Arm's length until she's in my arms, then what? After the gig we sat beside each other on wooden benches. Cold February wind making our cheeks flush. Arms tucked into our tummies. Legs crossed.

Buzzing off the night's events. Knees knocking. And then we kissed. Almost took me by surprise. Everything I wanted in one stretch. One movement, and I was lifted. Every skipped meal, every second I held my breath beneath the surface of my bath water, every time the phone rang out, every imaginary conversation, empty future, every walk through the graveyard, every extra-spicy Thai curry eaten without chewing, every friendly day out ruined – transcended. By the meeting of skin. I spread my wings and dived. Without a second thought.

*

Everything had been for this. Everything. Or had it?

Was it ever about this?

My heart still had a plaster on. Didn't want it ripped off. We had another honeymoon phase. High off rekindling. Back into the centre. But my time away from her was difficult to explain. She was the one who was betrayed after all. Can't have her pitying me. But the sense of abandonment was real. It will never not be real to me. And it doesn't make sense, or sit well morally. It corroded my insides. And, listen, this is the thing. In my mind, I've spoken and she's disappeared. Mouth open, door shut. That's what happened.

Someone I love disappeared because I said something. Because I did something wrong. Then pain. Little me's worst fear. Pulling up to broken trust in a new car has its challenges. Tuned engine or not. I had to prove I had both hands on the steering wheel. And I think I have. Transparency was key, to be begin with. Clarity on where

I was. No odd phone tactics. Passwords shared. All of that. Patience and understanding. And after the high I was more prepped for the bitter dip. The aftertaste. Until things flipped. Her shadow revealed itself. That, or she never truly forgave me. Upsurge of anxiety generally. Controlling behaviour. I struggled to implement boundaries. Guilt's only good once, as a reminder. But that's it.

I believe in energy. That our words carry weight. Even our thoughts play with the air surrounding us. We just don't have the instruments to measure that energy yet. I do believe that. And that truth is a compass. That piece I wrote in Brazil. The fact it resonated. Family have told me it's 'cause I was 'living in my truth'. I had connected to myself.

So what's really heartbreaking. For me anyway. Is that once we did reconnect. Chloe and me. Physically and emotionally. I was so scared of her leaving again that I began to lie. I started bending the truth. Omitting words and names. I couldn't bring myself to tell her how I'd got here. Just in case she didn't like it. I never betrayed her like that again but I betrayed myself a lot. The truth really does hurt.

What a sad way to keep someone from leaving me.

It's why I took in a rescue dog. A tale as old as time. A wagging tail for my mind. Love's a single word with countless complications. Doesn't make sense. Should be simple. Even though I'd dodged demons and done star jumps. I still held on to alone time like it was made of helium. I was trying my best, but love just wasn't simple enough. So one afternoon, in the middle of another cold spring, I responded to a message. One that had sat on my mind in a prayer pose.

'Do you want to rescue this dog? He's very intelligent. I think you'd get along.'

I love dogs. My dad used to have a dog and that dog was like my big brother. A big white Alsatian. Calm, loving and ethereal. Got a tattoo of him on my arm. Looked after a dog a few years ago too. A little French bulldog called Stanley. Couldn't fucking breathe. Snored constantly. Thought he was five times bigger than he was. Passed out if you laid him on his back. Only for a little while. Was a life saver, to be honest. And that memory lingered. How a dog can help a human reconnect. So I edged towards yes. Typed it. Sent it.

'Fantastic! I'll send through all the necessary details as soon as possible.'

The woman at the dog pound is called Bea. Bea's very efficient. A sniff of interest and you'd have a dog sooner than you thought. Very convincing. Did the work out of pure love. The pound was in Macedonia. They had to guarantee a certain number of adoptions before they could justify the twenty-six-hour drive. Bea had already convinced my mate of a new pup. So the process was faster than normal. Bea reckoned I was responsible enough to take on the challenge. And she promised that she would take the dog back herself if it didn't work out after three months.

So I waited. Stared at the three pictures they'd provided. Wondering if the dog was perfect or not. It's difficult to tell from a picture. Whether or not it's going to be the perfect dream scenario that should always happen. I projected my hope onto the Macedonian mutt. Hope that I could understand the simplicity of love. Chloe tried to get involved in the excitement. Bought a personalised dog collar. But I wasn't into it. Hated her involvement in fact. I needed this love all to myself. This was my choice, not hers. She had two cats. That was her thing. When the collar that she ordered arrived, I vibrated. She took the hint. Stepped back, let the bind tighten.

On the day of arrival, I received a phone call. 'Your dog is outside. Bring lead.'

Eastern European accent. No bullshit. I stepped outside. Caught the dog's eyes across the main road. The dog's ears pricked up as if he knew. My heart skipped. Waited till it was safe to cross. Woman handed me the dog, smiled, drove off. The dog rolled onto his back. Submissive. Scared perhaps. Lead on, the dog peed for what felt like five minutes. Was clearly disoriented. Nervous. Locked his legs a few times. Struggled to get through doorways. Eventually got into the flat. Lay down. Didn't move. Slept for thirteen hours.

I wanted to understand love in its purest form. Basic and reciprocal. Care for me, and I'll love you. I wanted to connect to my basic human responsibilities. And hope that they would reflect on myself and my immediate relationships. Also dogs forgive. Within reason. Which is a vibe. Still a flag though. That I wanted to keep Chloe away from him. Just in case. She had her cats. And those cats meant we had time apart. Which could have been keeping things together.

I guess her cats are fed now. But I savour these moments alone in the park. Tripping on shrooms. With my wonderful dog. My everyday connection to the universe. It hasn't been easy. Rebuilding a relationship after betrayal is tough.

Impossible for some. But we've given it a go. I couldn't do much more to prove my intentions. I'm still sober. And my ability to communicate has shifted a lot since The Bridge. I'm still in therapy. I look after my body. I'm doing the work. Sobriety is a big one though. I've never been a danger sober. I'm less risky without whisky.

*

Yes, you know this wolf.

So I'm a year into being back with Chloe. And I've been told I know this wolf by a woman in the dog park. That's what she's just said. Low cap now lifted. Holds my stare. That reply's halted me. I do know this wolf. I scan the fur and feel a tickle. The outline of a memory. And then I'm there, as a teenager, looking at this wolf.

Lorry.

Memorable dog name. Yes, I've heard the name before. As a teenager. I know this woman. Haven't seen her in around fifteen years. Her name's Mini. This is my dad's ex-girlfriend. Lorry is genuinely an eighth wolf. Almost illegal. Mini was with my dad for four years. And she has a daughter. Her daughter and I shifted from foot to foot and said 'hi' once. Spent an afternoon. Lorry was there. Mini says she's surprised we hadn't bumped into each other sooner, being that we live so close. I remember that I'm kind of tripping on mushrooms and decide not to say anything. Keep it moving. She asks which way I'm walking. She decides to walk the same way. Seems fair. I'm confident that her relationship with my dad didn't end well.

But I'm more open than usual, in a heightened state. She asks questions. As you do. The usual small talk, initially. Then we cut straight into it. It's quite shocking, the conversation, but I'm open. I usually am. The topic of partners arises. And I spill. Naturally. Why not? I say I'm back with a woman who left me. Mini says she always imagined me with her daughter, but her daughter thought that was weird because I'd be more like a brother. Then I think about the fact that I could have had a sister if my dad had been around more then. He'd spent more time with the other family than me during those four years. How bizarre.

When Mini asks more about my relationship situation she relives hers, seemingly. I mention that my girlfriend and I had been reading this book called *The Power of Now*. Mini puts her foot on the gas. Said her and my dad did the same thing. Starts to offload. No filter. I can't believe that they read the same book. A ray of sun breaks through the clouds. Like someone's looking for something. The discussion continues. I'm not attaching myself to any side but the parallels are hard to ignore. I'm certainly not taking her word over my dad's. I've heard from reliable sources she did some awful shit. But a few of these recollections of her time with my father are so familiar it's haunting. In present tense. Even with the high of shrooms. And these big green trees. How have I followed footprints I've never seen? Can a person inherit chaos?

Mini is a therapist. She says the love she had for my father was incredibly deep. Deeper than any love she'd felt before or since. But it began to feel like a descent. She found a core so cold she'd forget why she was even down there. Past a point, my dad was ice-cold. That's what she said. Not those exact words, but I'd had similar interactions with exes. Who felt confused as to why they were so drawn to me. And that I was impossible to hold. I was a firework display to them. Bright sparks and bangs until there's nothing left to light. Just darkness. And resistance. Some sentences are too bitter, too dazzling. She accuses my father of more stuff. Stuff best kept between the two of them. Or for my dad to tell me.

Like the fact my dad relapsed, at some point, on pain medication. Relapsed because my dad had previously been addicted to heroin. To opiates. Understandable, to be honest. But it did overlap with the beginning of my life. And, yeah, I wasn't allowed to see him for a bit. My mum never made him out to be a bad person. More clumsy than anything. Mini on the other hand . . .

It's quite telling that she's telling. Badmouthing a father to his son. I'm still listening with salt between my fingers. Surrounding trees still green and fuzzy. Overcast again. We leave the big field and circle back to the little park where we started. I come clean that I'd eaten a mushroom before this. She seems unfazed. She works with plants all of the time. Mini herself is only now experiencing a new relationship since the one with my dad. And as a therapist she deals with men in emotional crises all the time. Yeah, loads of unfaithful men who don't know whether or not to tell their wives. She's part of the brave team. Thinks I was brave to say something. She wants to put me back in touch with her daughter. And maybe have another dog walk. Back to the small park. Cap tilted back down and she's on her way home, Lorry by her side. I look at my own wolf and sit for a moment. Get my phone out and text Chloe. I tell her that the craziest shit just happened. And that I love her. And that I'm buzzing a little bit. But I'll explain when I see her. And then I'm with myself again. And I find myself conversing with a different wolf.

Mini aside, there were too many similarities. Mini was a menace, I know it. No angel. But regardless of the bullshit she might have stuck around it, I want to cut ties with that energy. Fuck this blueprint. Fuck this cycle. Got to switch it up. If there is any purpose worth fighting for, during my limited time on this earth, it's building a balanced child. Which is no easy feat. There's no such thing as a perfect parent. Everyone's trying their best. But I really would sit there. Awake. With my child. Present. That's the dream. Just to be there. Gravitational love. Up until three years old is the most important time. Then three to seven. Make it through those without too much chaos and you're good. Apparently. Fuck that up, and it's up to thirty years of remedial care. Heard that from Dr Gabor Maté. I can vouch for that. We don't all have to fold in on ourselves. There are other possibilities. Too many men have been consciously beaten and broken by the system that we're in. Families have been broken apart. It takes a village to raise a child, but that village needs men. All kinds of men. All ends of the spectrum but with connection to divinity intact. I want to hold my child's hand. Pick them up and point out my favourite constellation. Eat, sleep and sweep with them. Like how they did at that sacred house in Brazil. I want to laugh together. All of it. All of that pure, transcended energy.

The road feels narrower on the way back to my flat.

Cars moving faster. I can't make the same mistakes as my father. So I make a promise to myself that I will never leave the relationship that I'm in. I'll be on my knees in pieces before I give up. Even if my friends say that my face has changed. That I check my phone too much when I'm out. Feel a little panicked if she calls. I've got to know that I gave it my all. That I tried my hardest. That I didn't take the easy route.

35

The Right Kind of Anger

When I was little, I punched my mum in the stomach. I was fucking angry about something. Having to leave wherever I was. Didn't want to go. Or maybe I was just angry. But the memory troubles me. At the end of a corridor, daylight bleeding from rooms either side. But we're in the middle, in a prism of shadow. I'm at my auntie's and I don't want to leave. So I punch my mum in the stomach. And she folds like she's whispering to her knees. I've winded her. The woman who loves me and takes care of me. I've made it difficult for her to breathe. And this realisation fills me with regret and agony. I feel sick. Might as well have punched myself. A real punch in the gut. Guilt's a drain on the gut. It fills my body and reveals me. A reverse tip-and-strip pen. I'm clothed with a dark red guilt. On top of that, I'm not even in my body when I remember it. I'm down the corridor. Looking at the back of myself. Landing that blow. Wincing. Feeling sick.

Five years old. Reception. Primary school. North West London. Cafés springing up. Yummy mummy hotspots. Just up the road from the shop where I first had a piss

263

standing up, a framers called Worldly, Wicked and Wise. Break time and an older boy is giving me agg. We were playing three little pigs and it got out of hand. He was the wolf. He took it too far. Got physical. Threw me to the ground. Got filth all over my pale yellow jumper. Grey concrete all over my cotton. Called me a name and ran off. That day I was being picked up from school by my godmother. Tall, Middle Eastern, cheeky. Lived near a park full of dinosaurs. I told her about what had happened that day. That this wolf boy had pushed me over. She suggested that I go back in the next day and push him back harder.

Next day, I roll in. Waiting for the break. Anticipating my goal. Bell goes. Little legs on the painted lines. Hair ties and hopscotch. Kids running around headfirst. Legs trying to keep up. The boy's not in the same spot as yesterday. When I was a pig. So I go for a look out. I adventure into a newfound game zone. Same grey, different lines. Older kids. I notice the boy and he's wearing a hat. A loose-fitting hat that holds in the little locs he has. I take my opportunity and run over. I rip the hat off his head and hotfoot it. Adrenaline as gasoline. He can't catch me. Legs on smoke. Eventually a teacher intervenes. Then it's the end of the day and I'm being held back. Mum there. Teacher telling my mum what I'd done in the play-ground. Mum's frowning. She asks me why and I tell her what my godmother said. Her best friend. She silently acknowledges. Next time we all see each other, my mum makes her feelings clear. She says, 'Don't you ever teach my son to retaliate. That is not the kind of message I want him taking in at this age. He should never be encouraged to be violent, ok. It's bang out of order.'

She said it with some authority, I'll never forget it. And I felt bad. I started to believe that my anger was a bad thing. Ever since then my head often cools in confrontation. Which has its benefits in the moment. But in the long run the anger has to go somewhere. It's always got to go somewhere.

*

Driving through South London. In my first car. Nothing special. VW Polo. I pull up on a street with houses on the right and tennis courts on the left. Not fancy ones though. Rundown gravel tennis courts. Good-luck-trying-to-have-a-legitimate-tennis-career courts. I'm picking my friend up. He's visiting from LA for a month. We decide to get out of the city together. Escape to the sea and take stock.

Study mode. Energy from the waves. Silence at night. Just before I left, my mum mentioned something about a virus. Said a few people seemed to be freaking out on the news. Probably over the top though. Probably. Start of every zombie film. We get to the house out of the city by the sea. Settle in. Fish, chips and existential debate. Next day, national lockdown. The entire country freaked out and went still at exactly the same time. The world did. It was inconceivable. People panicked. I was sceptical. Head cooled as usual. Never trust the news anyway. Regardless, the system froze. We're kept inside for months. And during that first lockdown, I had a fucking great time.

Lockdown was the nail in the coffin for me and Chloe. For the best, as well. She had a very different approach to me. She panicked. I get why. A global unseeable threat was triggering for her, not particularly calming for her soul. We were holding on by a thread. By the last piece of pasta. Bound by duty and the fear of regret. Bound by the disbelief that a relationship so defined by sacrifice could lose its clarity. Surely not. After all this investment. After defying the odds. But the horse was dead. In the final month, Chloe got a new friend. Cool guy. Few years younger than me. The antithesis of me. And I felt a possibility. An escape route. Plus, Chloe would only waver if her heart had switched. I knew that. It was a relief. So in spite of my love for her cats and the holidays and the poems and the new friends and the fridge magnets and the butterflies and the gold-leaf personalised diary and the violins and the neighbours with the sweet child and the great café near hers and the Reebok Club classics and the games of Catan Universe – the door's closed. Chapter finished. For good reason. But it hurts. It still hurts. Still grief.

A different grief though. Because I knew I wanted out. So I watched the remnants of codependency play out in real time. My egoic desperation to reconnect with pain. Initially, we spoke. And danced in the deep zone. Performed. Reported our curated movements. Not wanting to appear too weak. But no one is above habit, and so much of the connection was habitual at that point. Two years. Two and a half if you count the hell gap. Zero contact was the only way. For a short period of time at least. Gabriella told me that, from experience. She said you have to block on social media and delete the number. It's the only way. That choice defied politics in that moment.

We live in a world where 'unfollowing' a human being is an attack. Blocking is unthinkable. Like it's beef or something. Right thing to do though. In the deep zone it's difficult to think straight. One thing I did know – confidently, with every fibre of my being – was that this ending would not break me.

We arranged to cease sound for a couple of weeks. No more good night or good morning. And I started to look after my body. I poured love into it. Half an hour of exercise every afternoon. Whole foods only. Made by me. Self-sufficiency. Every day felt like a love letter to my future self. This food will make me feel good. This sweat will keep me strong. There was a level of discipline. And I would walk my dog without my phone. Connect to wild flowers. Step into the breeze. Face up. Feel it. There was a point where I walked down to the beach one afternoon. A sunny afternoon. Empty shore. People in their houses. Ghost town other than the dog walkers. And this time it was just me. And the tide was out. Sliding away from us. My dog loves the water. Charges him. Whenever he walks in, he runs out. And I was completely with him. No podcast in my ear, no friends chatting, nothing. Felt lucky I wasn't in London. Shoes and socks off. Warm sand, cold water. Salt in the air. Seagulls in the air. No planes though. And we ran into the water. And then my dog ran out and grabbed one of my socks and started circling me. At full speed. Playing with the sock like it was an animal. He's usually so docile. This was full, uncensored joy. And I was full. Full to the brim. And felt grateful that the world had stopped. And like I was truly supposed to be there in that moment. Like I belonged there. And that sense of belonging is something I crave. Something I've always missed. A pool I've always tried to fill.

My gaze reaches the fold where the sun meets the sea. I feel stronger than I have done before. I'm going through it but I know I'll be ok. That's the difference. Awareness of the other side. I didn't have that a couple of years ago. That's the scariest part. Not knowing that there's a way out of it. And I wonder if that's why heartbreak can fuck men up to the extent that it does. If I'm anything to go by. Not only because we're really fucking sensitive, in spite of the denial, but because grief is something we can't fix. It's a fluid concept. A passing, wavelike emotion. And our avoidance of pain is noticeable. We've glamorised the coping mechanisms. Drinking, drugs, sex. The escape is accessible. Doesn't matter that we need pain to grow: we don't want to feel it.

We're used to more objective pain. Trauma that happens, then heals. Like getting punched in the face by a stranger. Or lifting a really heavy weight. Pain that can be measured with an expiry date, bandages, plasters. That kind of pain. Beyond that, we're in between stars. The darkness between diamonds. Reaching out, clutching at thin air, trying not to shift the atmosphere. Whereas women seem defined by pain. Have to roll with the punches for around a week a month. Touch death during birth. The world doesn't stop for them either. I think it should, but it doesn't. They have to carry on as usual. While their hormones fly around like tennis balls and their stomachs cramp. Uncontrollable. There's an element of surrender. An alien concept to me before. I just wanted the pain to stop.

I meant to say earlier, during that time, during that

broken heartbreak time, I went to a poetry night. At my worst. Good group. My writer friends. Poet, musician geniuses. A group I felt seen by. A group I'd go to France with to go to Afropunk and watch the World Cup final. Take photographs with. We were all at a poetry night at a university. One of the group was performing. Team was strong. Outside, we smoked. Four or five of us. Notably two women. One wonderful Caribbean woman, Keema, little fro, boyfriend in tow. Another African woman, Kez, with big locs, a sick jacket and the demeanour of a sage. She is a young sage. And because I'm in it, I talk it. Can't stop talking about how much the breakup was fucking me up. Asking if it's fair how I've been treated. If I did the right thing. If people would want to know if they'd been cheated on. Honestly, the group's divided. Some opting for self-preservation. Keema is totally on board with Chloe. The truth, yes, but also cheating, no, so bye bye. Others think it's harsh. One would never tell if they did. I'm searching for everything and anything I want to hear. Only the sentences to confirm the narrative I have in my own head. Can't stray from that. Too unnerving. Kez stayed quiet the whole time. Scanning for roots. I wanted her opinion badly. I respected her opinion. Eventually she breaks her silence.

She says, 'You can't let your past define you. I know you've been through a lot and there are reasons why you acted the way you did, why you're acting the way you are. But at some point you have to make a decision. You have to tell yourself that's not you any more.'

I had been obsessed with making it clear what I'd been through. Playing the victim. Focusing on the lack and blaming it for who I am now. Refusing to believe that somebody could not take it all into account. *I was abandoned! My dad's dealing with some dark shit! My mum hates herself!*

I basically eat my cigarette. Kez carries on: 'One day, you're going to wake up and you'll feel ok.'

*

So after agreeing not to talk for a couple of weeks, I imagine a world where Chloe hasn't taken up with that guy. And then another world where being told that she has doesn't affect me. Even though I'd wanted her to move on, the idea of them together still hurt. More because of the context than anything. Historic pandemic. I'm alone. We all have a certain duty of care to our partners when a breakup is mutual. That's what I believe anyway. The codependency reaches a new high. At night I find myself battling intrusive thoughts. Idealised images of Chloe. All my favourite parts of her edited into a highlight reel shown on repeat in the mind cinema. Invented explicitories of her and the new man. But my soul remains anchored. I knew I didn't want to be in the relationship. So in these moments I start training my brain to fight the images, to tie myself to the mast. My ego needs me to be in pain to be useful. So I push all the discontent to the surface. Memories of frowns, disappointment, restriction, clashing, tension, pursed lips. That curl on the outside of them when it's not going down how she wanted. Frowns have frowns sometimes. I made sure those images were replacing the idealised ones. Neuroplasticity. I actually fought the codependency. Rewired my brain. And it feels just the same. This feeling of breaking up with Chloe. As it did becoming sober. Relinquishing those desires. Some of my mates had a similar battle before doing a line of coke. Baggies out, remembering one night three months before where we had a good time. Overlooking the seventy-five other nights that we'd spent out since. Where fuck all happened. Just adrenaline and neglected pillows. Three to four days of regret. Seventy-two hours of imbalanced hormones and diluted chemicals. Improper decisions and self-loathing. But the ego wanted it. Same with lust or love or however we want to name it. I've come to terms with the part I had to play in the codependency too. Usually there's a dominant and a submissive role. And the sub has responsibility too. Mainly in holding their own boundaries. Boundaries are everything – boundaries meaning who and what we deem acceptable in our lives.

My authentic self is battling an unconscious, wounded version of myself and not losing. Huge for me. It's worth noting the undertone. The objectivity. In spite of how much we romanticise it, a lot of love comes down to choice. And our relationships are habit. Two things we can change.

Battle aside, the wound was real. We'd planned to be friends. To take it easy but keep the peace as a testament to our connection. Even engaging in a parting ritual. Do it properly. What a story. Now I feel betrayed, mugged off, frustrated. Envious even. What if I'm stuck on my own and she gets to fuck around with a new guy? Doting on her like a puppy. I started feeling as though Chloe would actually angle her phone away from me. Act cagey. Exactly the kind of behaviour she'd fear from me. But why do I feel like this if I'm over it? How can it hurt when I feel free? I start making moves in my head. Figure out which space I come off best. What makes me look great? The most powerful? The most chill? I figure I should forgive and move on. That's my play. Act like it's nothing. Like it's an everyday situation. Like walking the dog. And then she'll wonder why I'm so chill. And then I'll feel great. Forgiveness on toast, butter side up.

I call my therapist. Give her the lowdown. Communicate my play. First thing she says is: 'Don't forgive her yet.'

Which spins me out. Forgiveness is the bigger person. A giant move.

'Yes, but have you actually forgiven her?'

Semantics. Spanners. Do I want to hear this? No, I'm not sure if I've forgiven her.

'Just give it a moment.'

I give it a moment.

'Honestly, I think this is your golden ticket.'

Ears prick up. I'd love one of those. 'How so?'

'Because you're angry. And you're allowed to feel angry. And I think you'd do well to tap into that. You wanting to forgive might well be an attempt to control the situation. But emotions aren't rational. And you feel hurt. And you should honour that. Not worry about how the other person feels.'

'But I don't want her back or anything like that. If anything, I'm relieved. I should just drop it and move on.'

'Listen, if you want my advice, that's it. Don't forgive her. Allow yourself to feel angry. Ask yourself if you even want someone like that in your life.'

This conversation coincides with some nurturing Tai

advice. Some nurturing paternal fuckin' maternal whatever advice. He's checked on me nearly every day. On the phone. Asking if I'm cool. Same with Jake. They always show up when it matters. Tai kept questioning if I even need to have her in my life. What are the benefits for me? I said it's not about benefits, it's just good to be on good terms with exes. Is it? Maybe it isn't. And is it bad terms, really? Ideas were sprinkled into my psyche.

I listen to Chloe and wonder about morality. I wonder about what seems good or bad narratively. What it feels like to play the side I'm less used to. What other people's opinions on that would be. I decide to feign nonchalance. With a lump in my throat. Take it upon myself to do some more work. Write a couple of angry letters and burn them. Scream into a pillow. Start doing yoga. Keep up my high-intensity fitness training but make sure I film it and upload it online. I keep an altar. Practise gratitude. Give thanks. Smoke a thousand cigarettes, ring a thousand friends. Some cogs never left. And I must ask: have you ever been in a situation where your ex suggests that you take some time? To deal with the shock of their new relationship? Do they hope that you continue to be friends? Does the ex tell you that they love you? Those sacred words. I've learnt to cherish and value those words. There has to be respect in relationships. Respect and honest communication.

If you want to find out if someone's using you, tell them no. Tell them no and see how they respond. A person who respects you, your time and your boundaries will pass that no straight back with love. A gentle touch. New plan, no worries. A person who's using you will kick up a fuss. Centre themselves. Get frustrated. I've done it myself. Used to do it with Jake all the time. When he didn't want to come and chill with me when we were younger, I'd guilt-trip him into coming. Make a scene. Hold my hands up to it. Wouldn't do it now.

I decide I'm only going to communicate with Chloe using non-violent communication. Another special technique I learnt at The Bridge to ensure I wasn't catty. It's non-accusatory and direct. I can use it to explain why I don't want to be friends and what actions have taken place to encourage me to feel like that. It'll be great if she doesn't hit me back with an 'I'm sorry you feel that way' and ask me to drop her stuff off for her.

*

Not great. But now I'm free. Response felt chilly. Height of summer getting cold blows. Sat on my corner sofa. Heart racing. In disbelief. Confusion. Then cigarette. Then tears. Then rage. Then uncut anger. Anger that gives me the courage to stand up and face it all head-on. I ring all my close friends and say that I need them. I say I don't want contact with Chloe and it's done. A couple of them are all like, 'Ah, bro, but what if you end up getting back together and then I got to redo everything on socials?'

And I'm like, 'It's done. One hundred per cent. Trust me.'

Now I'm my own saviour. There's not a greater feeling. Fighting with both feet planted. Messages sent to the universe. Call and response. It's real. But I have to stay switched on. The greatest boxers are the best dodgers. And I always have myself to contend with.

I moan for a week. People ask me what I'm up to and I spill. Poor me. The nice guy for once. Having a time of it. It's funny being the funny one when it's not funny. Same extent, you find out your friends. The ones that check in. Hype you up. Tai and Jake like my left and right ear. And I was feeling myself. I'd become more attractive during my relationship with Chloe, I'm sure of it. I glowed up. More so in lockdown. My face, my hair. I'm stronger now. Used to dim it though. For real. Convinced myself I was blinding people. Or that I was blocking Chloe. I was in need of love that encouraged shining. When ready. Right now, still moaning. But every time I do, my chest tightens. And my tongue speeds up. Words falling out of my mouth. Can't help it. Need to tell everyone how shit the situation is. Until I read about emotional addiction. Online, actually. Wasn't even a book. It says emotion can become addictive too. That little pang of pain, shot of adrenaline, when recounting a story. And I realise. I've fallen into another cycle. Telling the same story, victimising myself, repeating myself. So I promise myself that I'll stay quiet. Zip my mouth from then. No more storytelling. And it's hard. Not filling silences. Not throwing words in the pot.

One morning when brushing my teeth I catch myself. As the brush thistles scratch at my enamel. Toothpaste dribbling off my lip. I catch my hypocrisy. I stare at my own audacity. To feel hard done by. Considering I've left more partners with this feeling, and worse, than I'd like to admit. I've said I love you, then betrayed them. More than once. Axed that trust. I've done it, man. Why am I holding a grudge? Don't need it. I completely understand why Chloe has acted the way she has. I properly get it. I would have done the exact same thing. Would have been difficult not to. Dimmer switch on full. I send the energies out there. Speak to some people. As a single man. And it feels good. But the process is different this time. I'm not looking to take anything, to conquer anyone. That's changed. I feel acutely aware of my own energy. Priorities weighted differently. I imagine how I'd feel in the presence of people. Who they know. What they do. How fluid our interactions would be. I'm online to pass the time, but we're in an age of mute messengers. Human beings who can make a keyboard sing but can't utter a single note in person. Yeah, pictures are nice. Angles are nice. Cool friends. But I value what I've got. I'm only exchanging sexual energy when I think it's worth it. When I know I need to. Value's just gone up. About eight years too late but we're here. Made a new playlist. I dance to it every morning. Dancing goes on the list. The love list. What I need from it.

*

This room's got a bed facing the window. I can sit up and see out. Proper sheets. One thing I never foresaw obsessing over. Thread count. Couple of pink pillowcases with unicorns on them. Bought for a joke. Now they make me happy. Head rested in the same position. On its side. Always outwards. Same pillow, different heads. Differing states of mind. I don't struggle with sleep. I'm lucky in that way. Never had a telly in my room. Always told myself stories till I disappear. Shut my eyes and imagine anything I want. Main character stuff. How I'd go about life events if I had powers. If I was a wizard. I've had phases of smoking weed before bed. When I used to be on my medication or I've had caffeine too late, I'd have a spliff. And I'd struggle with sleep sometimes then. But I don't often wake up in the night. Tonight I did. I can't be sure of the time.

Wasn't sure of the sound either. But I turned on my bedside lamp and my eyes confirmed it. My dog was howling. In his sleep. Eyes closed, in his dog bed, howling. Loud enough to wake me. He's never howled in waking life before. Not when music's on or if I do anything. I look straight out the window and it's a full moon. Swear on anything. The moon's beaming. Can't write this shit. Wolves howling at the moon's a myth apparently. Word is there's no 'evidence'. Something resonates. My calm, independent, loving, smart, docile, warm, beautiful black dog is a wolf at heart. I feel that.

36

Manuka

I'm introduced to someone new. Another mystery. It's not totally random. Years ago, and I mean years, a mate of mine mentioned that he thought 'you two would really get along'. Me and her. And at the time, I wasn't bothered. Distracted, I guess. But I'd noticed when sneaking around on the World Wide Web that this someone was single. So I say to my mate, what do you reckon? Still think we'd get along? Fancy pitching me to her? Didn't think much of it. Was kind of intrigued. Who knows? We're all stuck at home. Testing waters. He screenshotted my message and sent it. Straight to the point. She saw it. Found it funny, I guess. Messaged me. First bit done.

Thing is, after a couple of weeks I start rushing a bit. In my body. That high. We're messaging a lot. But I haven't been single that long so I try not to deep it. Just keep it moving. Not fight my urges, but be aware. I wanted to be very aware. Because I know how it can get. When that high blinds my judgement. Still, two weeks of us talking and I'm a little spun. I speak to Tai: he said he's not surprised. I speak to Jake: he said he thinks I'm ready. I was just with the wrong person before. He himself has had a quick change when he least expected it. It's like we synced up.

Refreshed. For the best. For everyone involved. And I wrote an actual list. Of what I wanted from love. Before speaking to her. I'd written a whole list. So that I could manifest the connection that I felt I deserved. Law of attraction. This quick though?

But I'm going down the list and she's ticked them all. Everything I wanted. Can't believe it. Like magic. We've spoken a few times on video now. But not in person. I've got to see if it's for real. I've got to feel her in my presence. We arrange to meet. I let my dog know. We're heading to a park around eighty miles away.

*

Now we're talking about anything. Finding a patch of grass that isn't lethal. Music, chatting, giggling. Whatever. All that shit. Kissed. It really works. Felt a bit like teen-agers. Eight hours melt into twenty minutes. Lipstick smudged. Dog's gone after squirrels. Who's the best Spice Girl? Detour under a tree. Still need a piss. Tentative goodbye at the car. Got a parking ticket.

*

We've been together two years and this relationship feels different. In the past I've been on edge. Rattled. A metal ball in a shaker. An escapist. One eye on the exit at all times. As if commitment was a turbo hoover, and I was just dust. On the cusp of removal. Now I've made a choice.

I've made that choice. Turned on a lamp. It's pleasant anticipation now. Loving her is like knowing the bread's warm. It's the half a second before I press play on my favourite record. It's a question in a quiz I know the answer to. Real talk. I know she's on my team. I believe that. I can see her heart from behind her as she walks alongside a friend of mine. Easy chat. No worries. Big family energy. I take in her outline. Her figure. Her stride. I've found a window in a stuffy room. I didn't know there was more space. It's a multi-sensory existential feeling. Gazing at her. Getting lost in transitions. Peaks of emotion. I really believe in her. I really believe that she's on my team. And she's a fucking warrior. I've watched her fight. The first thing she does every morning is smile. Sometimes she pees first. Great hugs. The shift into her fifth-gear grin. Nothing like it.

First time she came over to mine, we walked the dog together. Cool, late summer. Little jumper maybe. Thoughts flowing. Love bricks. Couple of years ago now. We sat down. Joked about. All of that shit. Came home. Made tea. She likes it strong. Says hailstones are just 'northern snow'. Hours later, I'd forgotten I'd booked an interview right when I was supposed to walk the dog. Before the light went. Can't have him off lead around foxes. Even if I love foxes. My dog doesn't care. I asked her if she could do it. She says 'yeah no worries'. Says she's going to leave her phone behind. I say 'cool' and jump into the interview.

Interview finished, I pop downstairs and she's not there. No sign of her or the dog. Twenty more minutes pass and a key pushes into the lock. Dog comes bouncing in. Tail flapping. She looks happy and spaced out. Space happy. Her vibe.

'You were gone for a while!'

'Oh, was I? Didn't even notice.'

'Was everything ok?'

'Yeah, I mean I've never walked a dog before but it was no bother.'

'You've never walked a dog?'

'No! So I just copied what you did.'

'Oh yeah? Off the lead. Everything?'

'Yeah. Is that not normal? I just walked up to the main grassy bit then took his lead off. He ran around for a bit and then came and lay down with me. Chilled out for a bit then we came home.'

'Wow. You're a natural.'

She is a natural. She's natural. I didn't respond for a second because I was just taking it all in. Dog's into her. So am I. I love her.

*

A couple of months later, we're apart. We're working separately. Nothing unusual. But longest yet.

I'm often distracted. I guess that's ADHD. My mind goes on adventures. If I open an app to respond to a message and there's another message that reminds me I haven't paid that fine that means I have to head downstairs but there's only one sock lying in the middle of the floor so I've got to find the other one until I see the kettle and reckon a cup of tea would help me finally sit down and start writing and then when I sit down I remember I have to walk the dog. Some days I'm more on top of it, some days not. Depending what's expected of me and when. It's a frustrating reality when dating, but every day I try my best. That day I wasn't good at responding. Not promptly anyway. We talk on the phone in the evening. My punctuality is not mentioned. I think it's all roses till she cuts off the call abruptly. Barely says 'I love you'. I'm shocked. I call back and ask what that was about. She explains that she felt ignored that day. I told her that if she began being passive-aggressive like that, my mind would begin to disintegrate. In the truest sense of the word. I laid it down as my boundary. If you have an issue with my behaviour, please make it clear directly. Withdrawal of affection will destroy me. I have to be clear. Even though I know it wasn't conscious and she didn't mean it that way. It was for the best of both of us. She understands. Agrees. And we move on. She didn't withdraw again. Pure love.

*

I still spiral. But less staircase, more spinning felt-tip pens. Whenever I feel a rupture, my go-to vices are low-key. And I welcome the spin. I have to. I am not perfect. Nobody is. I'm just trying to make the healthiest choices possible. And forgiving myself. For being born into such a chaotic shitshow. Full of beauty and wonder, no doubt. But a shitshow. There's more reflection than reflecting nowadays. We're tilted towards self-obsession but are part of a much bigger picture. A vast, universe-sized picture. And it's difficult to remember that. Because of all the words and pictures. All the numbers. So my current practice is to ride the moments that go beyond that. There are feelings that transcend language. Foreverness I can't do justice on paper.

Her smile is one of them. Her awe at the world is one of them. Her concern for others. I hope I get to experience it for a very long time.

*

My dad was rushed to the hospital a couple of weeks ago. He had pneumonia and was struggling to breathe. I was suddenly faced with his mortality and it shook me on a deeper level. It hurt. This man of mystery is going to disappear before I even got to ask him all my questions. Before I really find out what it was like being a black punk in the seventies. Before I get to hear about what he really felt like as a boy. A destabilising feeling. A collapsing pillar. It put everything into perspective. I knew it hit me on a deeper level because I started comfort eating. I ate cake and croissants, worrying about grief and what I'd missed. I went to see him in the hospital. He was hooked up to all these machines, some of them helping him to breathe. I sat with him and tried not to make any jokes, which was really difficult because that back and forth comprises a lot of our relationship. Making each other giggle. I just sat with him. He spoke to me more than he should have really. I just wanted him to rest. But he talks a lot about what's 'going on' these days. Not necessarily about how he feels. But just what he's thinking.

Honestly, I felt as though he was scared – something I've come to realise he hates admitting or being accused of. I notice a particular fight in him with any suggestion of how he's getting older or being unable to do certain things or having not fought his way to where is. He's proud. But maybe he'd even admit he was rattled by the ambulance. By the blue lights. He's got to kick the cigarettes now. Cut down from twenty a day. He said he's going to stop having sugar in his coffee. Be a little more health-conscious. But it appears the system isn't kind to those who stand against it. Live on the outskirts. Refuse to engage. And life's getting more tricky with age. But I'm here to support him. And my mum. Who continues to dazzle wherever she goes. If not a little pushy sometimes. Forever I hear about the feeling she gives people. That immediate lift. She honestly gets a kick out of helping people. I've said it before. Born warrior. Natural explorer. Been planning to 'sort her things out' for her entire life. Hoarder of pointless pieces of paper as well as love. My favourite moments in life now are when I see that light in their eyes. The glimmer and glint.

Light that's passed down. But I've grown aware that they won't be here forever. And that there's only so much I can do.

Now, when worry floats in my stomach, I can turn over in bed and ask a question to another soul I'm bound to. I can rest in that little nook between shoulder and neck. Often I'm provider, but when it's my turn I can't express the relief. The decompression. Being able to rest there even for five minutes. There's no height difference when we're lying down. There's no disparity at all when we're connecting emotionally. My girlfriend is entirely self-sufficient. Fucking hilarious, loving and kind. She's kind.

Listen, that's my advice. Find someone who's kind and makes you laugh. Easier said than done. But I can't knock her heart. I've knocked on it many a time and the door's always opened. An embrace is always an option. I really need it. Little things can still irritate me. Some days are hard. But on balance. On balance, my feet are touching the ground. I can feel my toes. And fucking hell, she deserves it. If anything, she can be too kind. Her heart is pure and warm and maybe my love has worth now. Maybe I'm good at loving someone now. And if I am, she deserves that. Because all she's done is work hard and help other people. And more shockingly, most of the time, I'm ok with her loving me. I can allow myself to believe that someone loves me a lot. That somebody wants to take care of me and wishes me the best. I believe it. It's such an odd feeling. I don't hear guys talk about it much. A foreverness. And I'm going to give it my all. Because even though love's hurt me before I'm not going to heal by running away from it. I'm meeting parts of myself I didn't know were there. I'm investing in a whole situation and it's fucking terrifying. But I'm here for it. I'm choosing to love. And with that support, I've never felt more like roaring. Growling, howling, whatever. I feel like I've died so many times.

And sometimes it's silence. I can sit with my partner for hours in silence. Walk through fields. Cross bridges. Seek refuge, in silence. As somebody who speaks so much, someone who hides in words, I've found it soothing. I've needed to calm the sentences down a bit. Not all the time. Sometimes. And in doing so, I've made space for the inexplicable. I want more people to know about love because it feels so much more embedded in the realms of existence than what we're fed daily. The endless narratives, hyperbole and escapism that pull us further away from ourselves.

My uncle in Brazil left me a voice note along these lines. I'll never forget it. Silence can allow for reconnection. And there have been moments when, looking into her eyes, being held by her, I've never felt more alive.

*

The wolf you feed. That so-called Native American proverb Tai recited to me many moons ago, was incomplete. In its filtered, internet-ready form, it's gone wayward. Only half the story. Turns out the story might have been created as part of a Christian sermon. Which makes sense in regard to the morality. Apparently in that version the wolves were 'white' and 'black' too. But it misses the point entirely.

You can't just feed one fucking wolf. Doesn't matter how full of joy, light and love the wolf is, life actually isn't that black and white. And, importantly, the other wolf will be fucking starving. Prowling your insides waiting for scraps or an opportunity to fuck the light wolf over. An unfed wolf won't disappear. It becomes more dangerous. And let's not pretend that our 'other wolves', our 'shadow wolves' or 'dark wolves', don't possess vital attributes. How are we meant to navigate this kind of world with light and love only? I don't believe it. That darker side got courage and tenacity. It can be fearless. And the opposing wolf is going to pop up one way or another. Goes without saying only feeding one wolf won't work. Ever. The truth is the wolves need to be by each other's side. Feeding both wolves maintains harmony. It honours the duality of our internal lives. It lessens the war within us. And that's the greatest win. Peace within. Can't be getting ripped apart by ourselves. Feed them right, feed the both.

So what about you? What wolf you been feeding lately?

Acknowledgements

It's important for me that I acknowledge the complexities of me even telling this story. I love writing. I always have done. These experiences were the first time I felt compelled to get something down in this form. In this format. And I've done so because I want to give people a chance. Pass along messages, teachings. I feel like that's what I'm here to do. But the story isn't pretty. It's one of growth, and people have been on the receiving end of my immaturity. Who have had to deal with themselves through different means. Just get on with it. Not make the same mistakes. I wish I was on good terms with everyone, but I'm not. Sometimes life goes like that. I've learnt that. But I acknowledge that I have some balance to restore.

J. In spite of you receiving the best version of me to date (not perfect), it's still not easy reading about my past relationships. I told you from the very beginning that I was only able to look back and dissect now I felt safe, and you believed me. Not only that, you were patient and kind and you read my drafts and just told me all of the bits that you loved and continued to understand my aim.

You've been so supportive, you're a beautiful human being and I love you.

My agent, Zoe. Again, patience, I can't thank you enough. There were years between an approach for me to write a book and an actual proposal coming into fruition. The second I was ready, so were you. And you helped me maintain focus even when I was sending you random side missions and wildly tangential streams of consciousness. On top of that. Imposter syndrome, paranoia. I'll always try and keep this shit in therapy but the career-based stuff does slip out. You also encouraged me to double down on my style of writing which has been huge for me as a writer. It dislodged a whole block I didn't even realise I had. I hate commas. You let me know that was ok. Now look at us.

Francis. Had no idea we'd end up working together when I bumped into you and Jamie on Portobello. But you've been a rock. An anchor. Especially in these latter stages. I've messaged you at completely unacceptable times. And you've calmed me. Fuck me, I've spiralled a lot. I will forever appreciate your time and smile and belief and patience and love of dogs and people and Edinburgh. Busy and still present. Thank you. Melissa too. Invaluable guidance when my compass was fucking everywhere. Thank you for your honesty and awareness and notes and affirmations. Feel blessed for real. Jamie. You had already welcomed me into a surrogate family before this whole book shit came about. Felt right. I'm glad it's worked out this way. Unwavering support. Your gifts are stacked. Big up Canongate.

Honourable mention to my therapist. Saved my life a bit, to be honest. She knows. See you soon. Donna Lancaster. I have to put your full name so people look you up. I don't even have the words. I'm just so glad you reached out. Again, wouldn't be here without you. You have an immovable belief in me which I struggle to really comprehend sometimes but that's all part of the work. I just want everyone to know you so that they can be moved too. Gabby and Freddie. Everyone at The Bridge. I could have just written the book about that experience. I hope it returns one day.

Adam, thank you for sitting down with me in a park and showing me how to build structure. Without the scaffolding to this book I wouldn't have been able to write it. And the techniques and guidance you showed me that afternoon have stayed with me ever since. You're an incredible playwright and generous with your expertise. You deserve all the credit. Johann. Mate. Without you I wouldn't have met Zoe or Jamie or Rebecca. You read my article and told me that I could write a book. And not only that you helped me do it. You made huge introductions for me selflessly. And checked in on how I was doing. Fuckin' insane. All while you were off on your own unfathomable investigations. I was well excited to tell you I'd actually got round to writing it. These thank yous aren't in order. Thank you Caleb for the body doubling and inspiration. Joshy, Mak, Harley, Flynn, Charlotte, Charley, Iona, Charlie, Ayishat, Iggy, Lex, Karina, Lola, Holly, Jack P, Sam, Ben, Bleue, Pete C, Tommy D and the fam for being in and around the rebuild. Coarse way of putting it but you know what I mean. Huge parts of my life. Even though all I do is walk my dogs these days. I won't forget. Trev. Lockdown. Unforgettable. Endless everything. Core and conversation. Thandie and Kay. Massively supportive. Dolly, what a legend. I called you with concern when I first started and you talked me through it. Have been on hand ever since. Been tough and you've been there. Thank you. Afua. My first proper reader. I was lost in my own fear before you sent me those messages. Infinite love. My beautiful family. Splintered but sacred. Special. There more than I realise. Sita, Hannah, Eddie, Richard, Liz. Found family. The tribe. Honestly I was fluttering around everywhere. All these interactions mean so much to me. Of course, my mum and dad. I appreciate you and love you. Forever.